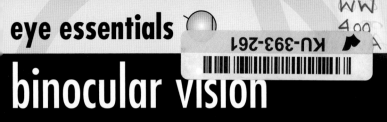

eye essentials

binocular vision

Bruce Evans PhD, FCOptom, DipCLP, DipOrth, FAAO
Director of Research, Institute of Optometry, London, UK
Visiting Professor, City University, London, UK
Examiner in Binocular Vision and Diploma in Orthoptics syllabus co-author,
College of Optometrists, UK

SERIES EDITORS

Sandip Doshi PhD, MCOptom
Optometrist in private practice, Hove, East Sussex, UK
Examiner, College of Optometrists, London, UK
Formerly Clinical Editor, Optician

William Harvey MCOptom
Visiting Clinician and Director of Visual Impairment Clinic,
City University, London, UK
Professional Programme Tutor for Boots Opticians Ltd
Clinical Editor, Optician, Reed Business Information, Sutton, UK

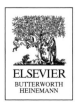

ELSEVIER
BUTTERWORTH
HEINEMANN

EDINBURGH LONDON NEW YORK OXFORD
PHILADELPHIA ST LOUIS SYDNEY TORONTO 2005

ELSEVIER
BUTTERWORTH
HEINEMANN

© 2005, Elsevier Limited. All rights reserved.
First published 2005

No part of this publication may be reproduced, stored in a retrieval system, or
transmitted in any form or by any means, electronic, mechanical, photocopying,
recording or otherwise, without either the prior permission of the publishers or a
licence permitting restricted copying in the United Kingdom issued by the
Copyright Licensing Agency, 90 Tottenham Court Road, London W1T 4LP.
Permissions may be sought directly from Elsevier's Health Sciences Rights
Department in Philadelphia, USA: (+1) 215 238 7869, fax: (+1) 215 238 2239,
e-mail: healthpermissions@elsevier.com. You may also complete your request
on-line via the Elsevier homepage (http://www.elsevier.com), by selecting
'Customer Support' and then 'Obtaining Permissions'.

ISBN 0 7506 8850 5

British Library Cataloguing in Publication Data
A catalogue record for this book is available from the British Library.

Library of Congress Cataloging in Publication Data
A catalog record for this book is available from the Library of Congress.

Note
Knowledge and best practice in this field are constantly changing. As new research
and experience broaden our knowledge, changes in practice, treatment and drug
therapy may become necessary or appropriate. Readers are advised to check the
most current information provided (i) on procedures featured or (ii) by the
manufacturer of each product to be administered, to verify the recommended
dose or formula, the method and duration of administration, and
contraindications. It is the responsibility of the practitioner, relying on their own
experience and knowledge of the patient, to make diagnoses, to determine
dosages and the best treatment for each individual patient, and to take all
appropriate safety precautions. To the fullest extent of the law, neither the
publisher nor the editors assumes any liability for any injury and/or damage to
persons or property arising from this publication.

Working together to grow
libraries in developing countries
www.elsevier.com | www.bookaid.org | www.sabre.org

ELSEVIER   BOOK AID
             International   Sabre Foundation

ELSEVIER   your source for books,
journals and multimedia
in the health sciences

www.elsevierhealth.com

Printed in China

The
publisher's
policy is to use
paper manufactured
from sustainable forests

Contents

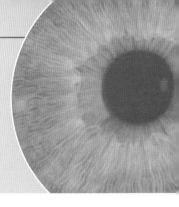

Preface

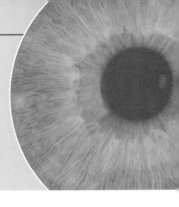

Orthoptics (binocular vision anomalies) is not an optional subject for primary eyecare practitioners (typically, optometrists). Most patients have two eyes and eyecare practitioners must therefore be able to at least recognize binocular vision anomalies and to treat, correct, or refer as appropriate. Yet discussion with optometrists and ophthalmologists, whether newly qualified or experienced, suggests that orthoptics is often a subject with which these professionals feel ill at ease.

There are now quite a considerable number of textbooks available on orthoptic or binocular vision anomalies. Most of these books seem to have been written with the specialist practitioner in mind and tend to contain enough detail to take a practitioner from the level of newly qualified up to that of an expert in the field. Yet, it has to be acknowledged that only a small proportion of eyecare practitioners are interested enough in orthoptics to wish to specialize in this field. Many eyecare practitioners just wish to know enough about this subject to practice in a competent and safe way. I have written this book for these practitioners. I have tried to concentrate on the basic information that practitioners need to know, with strong emphasis on "hands on" clinical methods. The main orthoptic tests are described in boxes that give a simple, step by step, guide on how to carry out the test and to interpret the results. There are many figures to illustrate these tests and other clinical observations.

I spend most of my working week practising in a community eyecare practice and the book concentrates on the conditions and issues that are most likely to be encountered in this setting. I hope that this book might live near the kettle for browsing! I also hope that the "ready reference layout" will mean that practitioners are able to quickly look up a test or condition.

I also hope that the book will be useful for students of optometry, orthoptics, and medicine. The many tables and simple test descriptions should be especially useful to those who are revising for examinations.

Many of the techniques and theories described in this book are elaborated on in greater detail in Pickwell's Binocular Vision Anomalies, 4th edition by BJW Evans.

Further reading

Evans, B.J.W. and Doshi, S. (2001). Binocular Vision and Orthoptics. Butterworth-Heinemann: Oxford.

Evans, B.J.W. (2002). Pickwell's Binocular Vision Anomalies. Butterworth-Heinemann: Oxford.

Evans, B. (2004). The Diploma in Orthoptics. Part 1: A "how to" guide. *Optician* **226**, 26–27.

Noorden, G.K.V. and Campos, E. (2002). Binocular Vision and Ocular Motility: Theory and Management of Strabismus. Mosby: St Louis.

Rabbetts, R. B. (2000). Bennett & Rabbetts' Clinical Visual Optics. Butterworth: Oxford.

Rosenbaum, A.L. and Santiago, A. P. (1999). Clinical Strabismus Management. W.B. Saunders & Company: Philadelphia.

Foreword by series editors

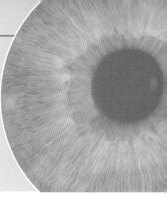

Eye Essentials is a series of books intended to cover the core skills required by the eye care practitioner in general and/or specialized practice. It consists of books covering a wide range of topics, ranging from: routine eye examination to assessment and management of low vision; assessment and investigative techniques to digital imaging; case reports and law to contact lenses.

Authors known for their interest and expertise in their particular subject have contributed books to this series. The reader will know many of them, as they have published widely within their respective fields. Each author has addressed key topics in their subject in a practical rather than theoretical approach, hence each book has a particular relevance to everyday practice.

Each book in the series follows a similar format and has been designed to enable the reader to ascertain information easily and quickly. Each chapter has been produced in a user-friendly format, thus providing the reader with a rapid-reference book that is easy to use in the consulting room or in the practitioner's free time.

Optometry and dispensing optics are continually developing professions, with the emphasis in each being redefined as we learn more from research and as technology stamps its mark. The *Eye Essentials* series is particularly relevant to the practitioner's requirements and as such will appeal to students, graduates sitting professional examinations and qualified practitioners alike. We hope you enjoy reading these books as much as we have enjoyed producing them.

Sandip Doshi

Bill Harvey

Acknowledgment

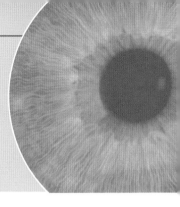

I am grateful to Louise Williams and Simon Harris for their helpful comments on the manuscript.

1

Overview of binocular vision anomalies

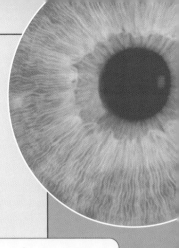

What are binocular vision anomalies?

Binocular vision anomalies occur when there is a problem in the co-ordinated use of the eyes as a pair. Inevitably, the prevalence of binocular vision anomalies varies according to the precise criteria that are used to define these conditions. A conservative estimate is that binocular vision anomalies affect 5% of patients consulting primary eyecare practitioners.

The classification of binocular vision anomalies starts with two fundamental distinctions, summarized in Figure 1.1. One distinction is comitant/incomitant and the other is strabismic/heterophoric. These two approaches to classification are complementary, not exclusive. For example, comitant

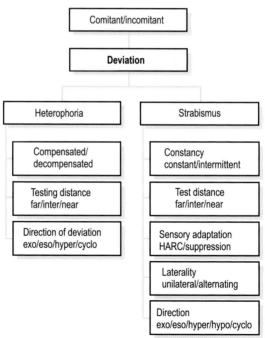

Figure 1.1 Classification of binocular vision anomalies

deviations may be strabismic or heterophoric and strabismic conditions may be comitant or incomitant.

Incomitancy (Chapter 6) is defined as a deviation that varies in different positions of gaze and that varies depending on which eye is fixing. Incomitant deviations affect about 0.5% of the population.

A strabismus (Chapter 3), also known as a heterotropia or squint, occurs when the visual axes are deviated: where the line of sight of one of the eyes does not fall on the object of regard. Strabismus affects around 2.5–4% of the population. A strabismus can be constant or intermittent, and can be unilateral or alternating. Young patients develop sensory adaptations to a strabismus, typically harmonious anomalous retinal correspondence (HARC) or suppression (see p. 42).

Most people do not have a strabismus and the eyes are kept in perfect, or very close to perfect, alignment. But when one eye is covered, or the two eyes are dissociated (prevented from viewing the same scene), most people develop a latent deviation (heterophoria). A heterophoria (Chapter 2) is a normal finding: it is only apparent when the eyes are dissociated and is not present under normal viewing conditions. Occasionally, a heterophoria may decompensate, when it can cause symptoms and in some cases might break down into a strabismus. As well as being classified as compensated or decompensated, a heterophoria can also be classified according to the testing distance.

Both strabismus and heterophoria can be classified according to the direction of the deviation: eso for when the visual axes turn inwards, exo for outwards, hyper for upwards, hypo for downwards, cyclo for cyclorotation. Heterophoria is sometimes described as a latent strabismus, but this term can be confusing since a heterophoria is a normal finding which is usually not a cause for concern.

How do I investigate?

Symptoms and history are crucial to the investigation of binocular vision anomalies, and the symptoms of decompensated heterophoria are listed in Table 2.1. Most children with strabismus do not report symptoms, so parents should be asked whether an eye ever appears to "wander" or "turn". Family history is also important, especially with child patients. Parents should be asked if there is any family history of a "turning eye", "lazy eye", poor vision, or of refractive error (particularly long-sightedness). A family history of any of these will increase the risk of a strabismus being present.

One commonly asked question about orthoptic tests is "Should the patient wear a refractive correction?" For nearly all orthoptic tests, the answer is the same: the patient should wear any refractive correction that they usually wear for tasks at that distance. If there is reason for concern over binocular co-ordination and the practitioner is considering prescribing a refractive correction that is significantly different to that which is already worn, then the relevant orthoptic tests should be repeated with the new prescription in place.

Most orthoptic investigative techniques will be described in the relevant sections of this book. However, one orthoptic test is at the very core of the investigation of a great many binocular vision anomalies and will be described here: the cover test. Like most other orthoptic tests, it should be repeated at the key distances at which the patient works.

The cover test

Typically, the cover test (Figures 1.2 and 1.3) is carried out using as a target a letter from the line above the worst eye's visual acuity. If the visual acuity is worse than 6/60 then a spotlight can be used. If the eye examination results in a significantly different prescription to that previously being worn then the cover test should be repeated with the proposed new prescription in place.

Often, the patient's history or previous records lead the practitioner to suspect that a strabismus may be found in one eye, which is likely to be the eye with the worse acuity. If so, then the other eye should be covered first. This first cover is the "purest" orthoptic test of all, since the moment before the cover is applied the patient has normal binocular vision and is viewing the target in a completely natural way. The eyes should be

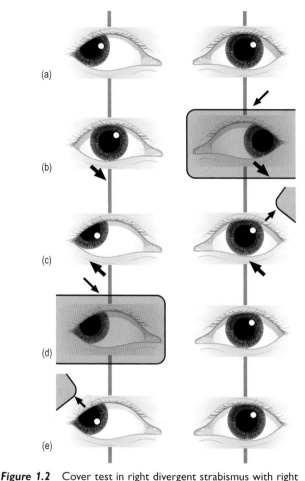

Figure 1.2 Cover test in right divergent strabismus with right hypertropia (movement of the eye is signified by the solid arrow, movement of the cover by the dotted arrow): (a) right eye deviated out and up; (b) left eye covered – both eyes move left and downwards so that the right eye takes up fixation; (c) left eye uncovered – both eyes move right and upwards so that the left eye again takes up fixation; (d) and (e) no movement of either eye as the strabismic right eye is covered and uncovered. See text for explanation (reproduced with permission from Evans, B.J.W. (2002) *Pickwell's Binocular Vision Anomalies*, 4th edition, Butterworth-Heinemann)

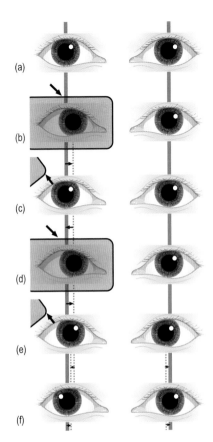

Figure 1.3 Cover test in esophoria (movement of the eye is signified by the solid arrow, movement of the cover by the dotted arrow): (a)–(c) from the 'straight' active position, the right eye moves inwards when dissociated by covering (b); it moves smoothly outwards to resume fixation with the other eye when the cover is removed (c). Note that the left (uncovered) eye does not move during the 'simple pattern' of movements (d)–(f). The "versional pattern": the right eye moves inwards under the cover, as in the simple pattern (d); on removing the cover, both eyes move to the right by the same amount (about half degree of the esophoria) (e); both eyes diverge to the straight position (f) (reproduced with permission from Evans, B.J.W. (2002) *Pickwell's Binocular Vision Anomalies*, 4th edition, Butterworth-Heinemann). See text for explanation.

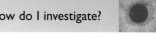

watched as the cover approaches since if a dissociated vertical deviation (p. 56) is present then a movement of an eye is often seen before the cover actually reaches the eye.

The use of the cover/uncover test to detect strabismus is described in Table 1.1, and its use to detect heterophoria is described in Table 1.2. It is useful to estimate the angle of any eye movements, and a method for this is described in Table 1.3. In

Table 1.1   Detection of strabismus with the cover/uncover test

1. As the cover moves over one eye then the practitioner should watch the uncovered eye. It is the behavior of the uncovered eye that reveals whether the patient has a strabismus

2. For example, as the left eye is covered the practitioner should watch the right eye. If the right eye moves then this suggests that there is a strabismus in this eye (Figure 1.2, the behavior of the right eye from (a) to (b))

3. The direction and amplitude of the movement should be estimated (see Table 1.3)

4. The cover is then slowly removed from the eye that has been covered and this eye is observed to see if a movement occurs, signifying heterophoria (see Table 1.2)

Table 1.2   Detection of heterophoria with the cover/uncover test

1. As the cover is slowly removed from the eye that has been covered then this eye is observed to see if a movement occurs. If a movement occurs as an eye regains fixation after being covered then this indicates a heterophoria (e.g., in Figure 1.2 the right eye moves out as the cover is removed from (b) to (c))

2. The direction and amplitude (Table 1.3) of the movement should be estimated

3. The quality of this recovery movement should also be recorded. This gives an objective indication of how well the patient is able to compensate for the heterophoria (Table 1.4). A higher grading in Table 1.4 is more likely to be associated with decompensation and thus more likely to require treatment

Table 1.3 Estimating the amplitude of movement on cover testing

1. The amplitude of movement should always be estimated (in Δ) and recorded during cover testing
2. It is easy to train yourself to be quite accurate at this, and to regularly "calibrate" your estimations. On a typical Snellen chart, the distance from a letter on one end of the 6/12 line to a letter on the other end is about 12 cm (measure this on your chart to check). If the distance is 12 cm, this means that when the patient changes their fixation between these two letters the eyes make a saccade of 2Δ (1Δ is equivalent to 1 cm at 1 m)
3. If you place two markings on the wall near the letter chart that are 24 cm apart, when the patient changes their fixation between these two marks then the eyes are moving by 4Δ
4. After you have done the cover test and estimated the amplitude (in Δ) of the strabismic or heterophoric movement, remove the cover and have the patient look between these two marks, or between the two letters on the 6/12 line whilst you watch their eyes. Compare the amplitude of this eye movement with the amplitude of movement that you saw during cover testing, to check the accuracy of your estimate
5. A similar method can be used for larger amplitudes
6. At near, this task is even easier. Use as your fixation target the numbers on a centimeter ruler which you hold at $1/3$ m. If the patient looks from the 1 to the 2 then the patient's eyes are moving by 1 cm which, at $1/3$ m, equates to 3Δ

heterophoria, the quality of recovery movement should also be quantified, and a grading system for this is described in Table 1.4.

The description above is of one form of the cover test: the **cover/uncover test**. This is useful for detecting strabismus, for estimating the magnitude of the deviation under normal viewing conditions (Table 1.3), and for evaluating the recovery movement in heterophoria (Table 1.4). But it is also useful to know how much the angle increases ("builds") as the patient is dissociated to greater degrees by alternate covering. So, after the

Table 1.4   A grading system that can be used to gauge cover test recovery in heterophoria

Grade	Description
1	Rapid and smooth
2	Slightly slow/jerky
3	Definitely slow/jerky but not breaking down
4	Slow/jerky and breaks down with repeat covering, or only recovers after a blink
5	Breaks down readily after 1–3 covers

cover/uncover test it is advisable to alternate the cover from one eye to the other for about six further covers to see how the angle changes (Table 1.3). At the end of this **alternating cover test** as the cover is removed then the recovery movement can be observed again to estimate the effect of alternate covering on the recovery (Table 1.4). A cover/uncover test is then performed once more on the other eye to assess any change in the recovery of this eye. An example of the recording of cover test results for a patient is given in Table 1.5.

Table 1.5   Example of a recording of cover test results

D 2Δ XOP G1 → 2Δ XOP G2
N 8Δ XOP G1 → 12Δ XOP G3
Key: at distance, the cover/uncover test reveals 2Δ exophoria with good (grade 1) recovery. After the alternating cover test the angle does not change but the recovery becomes a little slower (grade 2 recovery)
At near, the cover/uncover test reveals 8Δ exophoria with good recovery. After the alternating cover test the angle builds to 12Δ exophoria with quite poor recovery, but not quite breaking down into a strabismus (grade 3 recovery)

A great deal of information can be gleaned from the cover test. Table 1.6 includes some additional comments. Other methods of assessing ocular alignment are available, including the Hirschberg and Krimsky tests which are based on an observation of corneal reflexes. But these tests are inaccurate. With practice, cover testing is nearly always possible, even with infants.

Table 1.6 Additional comments on cover testing

- With the alternating cover test, as the angle **builds** towards the **total angle**, it becomes easier to detect vertical deviations which are typically smaller than horizontal deviations

- Vertical deviations also can sometimes be spotted by watching for movement of the eyelids

- In some patients, an eye is deviated before the test (strabismus) or becomes deviated during the test and is very slow to take up fixation. So, when the dominant eye is covered there may be no apparent movement, even though the uncovered eye is not fixating the target. A movement of the deviated eye can sometimes be elicited by asking the patient to "look directly" at the target, or by moving the fixation target a little

- The magnitude of the deviation can also be measured using a prism bar or loose prisms, typically during the alternating cover test. This is especially useful in large angles where accurate estimations of angular movements becomes difficult

When do I need to do something?

As a general rule, there are only three reasons for intervening when a binocular vision anomaly is present. These are listed in Table 1.7.

It should be noted that not all patients with symptoms are aware of their symptoms. This is especially true of children who may only appreciate that a symptom was present once the condition has been successfully treated. It is only very rarely that binocular vision anomalies are encountered in primary eyecare practice which result from ocular or systemic pathology, but the practitioner should always be alert to this possibility.

Table 1.7 **Reasons for intervening when a binocular vision anomaly is present**

1. If the anomaly is causing symptoms or decreased visual function
2. If the anomaly is likely to worsen if left untreated
3. If the anomaly is likely to be a sign of ocular or systemic pathology

Occasionally, heterophoria is encountered which may be in the process of breaking down to a strabismus yet the patient may have a sensory adaptation (e.g., suppression) so that they do not have any symptoms. This is an example of a condition that is likely to worsen (become a strabismus) if left untreated.

Figure 1.4 is a simple model of binocular vision anomalies affecting fusion and is useful for considering what happens when people develop fusional problems and what approaches might be appropriate for treatment. When an eye is covered (dissociated) most people will exhibit a dissociated deviation. Hopefully, during normal binocular fixation the person can overcome this dissociated deviation to render it compensated. Three factors influence how easy it is for a person to overcome their dissociated deviation. First, the size of the dissociated deviation is

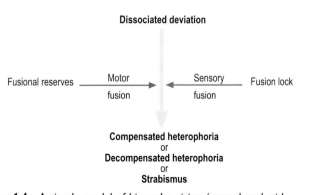

Figure 1.4 A simple model of binocular vision (reproduced with permission from Evans, B.J.W. (2002) *Pickwell's Binocular Vision Anomalies*, 4th edition, Butterworth-Heinemann)

of some relevance: if it is very large then it is likely to be harder for the person to overcome it. A second factor is the force of motor fusion, which can be measured as the fusional reserves (Figure 1.4). A person with a heterophoria constantly exerts motor fusion to overcome their heterophoria, so their fusional reserves have to be adequate. Some conditions (e.g., illness, stress, old age) can cause the fusional reserves to deteriorate resulting in a previously compensated heterophoria decompensating. This explains some cases where a childhood illness causes a heterophoria to break down into a strabismus.

The third factor that influences how well a person can overcome their dissociated deviation is sensory fusion (Figure 1.4). This relates to the similarity of each eye's image. For example, a person may have a compensated heterophoria until they develop a degraded image (e.g., from refractive error, age-related cataract, macula degeneration), when each eye's image become less similar. This impairment of sensory fusion causes their heterophoria to decompensate.

When a patient presents with a decompensating heterophoria then a consideration of Figure 1.4 will usually enable the cause of decompensation to be determined. If the dissociated deviation has changed, then the reason must be determined: a large change in dissociated deviation might be a sign of pathology.

If a non-pathological reason for decompensation can be found then the alleviation of this could render the patient compensated. One treatment might be to strengthen motor fusion by training the fusional reserves. In a case of anisometropia (which impairs sensory fusion through aniseikonia), a treatment might be to prescribe contact lenses to equalize the retinal image size.

What do I do?

When binocular vision anomalies require an intervention then there are several possible options:

1. treat with eye exercises
2. treat with refractive modification

3. treat with prisms
4. treat with patching (occlusion) or penalization
5. refer for one of the above treatments by another practitioner
6. refer for surgery
7. refer for further investigation.

These options are not mutually exclusive. For example, a child with strabismic amblyopia where the cause of the strabismus is not clear may be referred for medical investigation, but whilst waiting for the hospital appointment the primary eyecare practitioner can start patching. As in all healthcare sciences, the diagnosis and management are not fixed entities, but rather are the latest judgments based on the best available evidence at that time. Very often, one treatment is tried in the first instance and if this is not effective then a second-choice treatment will be tried. Practitioners should always try to keep an open mind about their diagnosis and should be prepared to constantly reconsider this in light of their latest findings and of the patient's response to any treatment.

2
Heterophoria

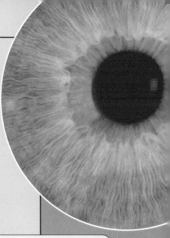

What is heterophoria?

Heterophoria is a tendency for the eyes to move out of alignment when one is covered or when they view dissimilar objects. Types of heterophoria are **exophoria**, **esophoria**, **hyperphoria**, and **cyclophoria** (see pp. 2–3). Some authors used to call a heterophoria a "latent strabismus" or "latent squint".

One way of thinking about heterophoria is to consider the resting position of the vergence system. In total darkness the eyes adopt a resting position (tonic vergence) where, for most people, they align on an imaginary object about 1–2 m away. Distance vision can be thought as requiring divergence away from this resting position and similarly near vision requires convergence away from this resting position. When one eye is covered, that eye is dissociated and tends to revert towards the resting position. That reversion is the heterophoria. Typically, the heterophoria is visualized during the cover test when the cover is removed and the eye re-aligns to take up fixation. This way of thinking about heterophoria in terms of the typical resting position explains why most people have a small esophoria for distance fixation and a slightly larger exophoria at near.

How do I investigate?

Symptoms

Symptoms are important in determining whether a heterophoria is decompensating. Typical symptoms that may be present in decompensated heterophoria are listed in Table 2.1. It was noted on p. 10 that some patients do not appreciate that they have symptoms until these have been corrected. Occasionally, patients may not have symptoms from a decompensating heterophoria because they develop a **sensory adaptation** (e.g., foveal suppression; see below). Additionally, many of the symptoms in Table 2.1 are non-specific: they could result from other, non-orthoptic, causes. So clinical tests are necessary to determine whether any symptoms are likely to result from an orthoptic problem and therefore to be treatable by orthoptic means. These tests are described below.

Table 2.1 **Symptoms of decompensated heterophoria**

Number	Type of symptom	Symptom
1	Visual	Blurred vision
2		Double vision
3		Distorted vision
4	Binocular	Difficulty with stereopsis
5		Monocular comfort
6		Difficulty changing focus
7	Asthenopic	Headache
8		Aching eyes
9		Sore eyes
10	Referred	General irritation

Cover test recovery

In young children or uncooperative older patients (e.g., patients with intellectual impairment), objective testing may be required to determine if a heterophoria is decompensating. An assessment of cover test recovery can be extremely important in these cases, as described on pp. 7–9.

Mallett fixation disparity test (aligning prism)

The Mallett fixation disparity test is an extremely valuable test for assessing heterophoria. The distinction between strabismus, when the visual axes are misaligned, and heterophoria, when the visual axes are aligned unless the patient is dissociated, is in fact not as clear-cut as might be thought. There needs to be some 'free play' in the visual system so that the eyes can move slightly out of alignment during normal binocular vision, for example during a large saccade. This free play is made possible because of Panum's fusional areas: there are matching areas on each retina that correspond rather than points. So, there can be a minute misalignment (**fixation disparity**) of the visual axes without the patient suffering diplopia or strabismus. This misalignment is small, typically a few minutes of arc, and is less than the deviation of the visual axes that is present in strabismus.

Although fixation disparity occurs without the patient suffering diplopia, it is still undesirable. It causes a reduction in stereo-acuity and (when using well-designed fixation disparity tests) indicates that the visual system is under stress (see Figure 1.4). As Figure 1.4 shows, sensory fusion is very important in helping a patient to keep a heterophoria compensated. Under normal viewing conditions, the majority of the field of view is seen by both eyes and acts as a **fusion lock**. In any fixation disparity test, a small section of visual field must be excluded from the fusion lock: these are the monocular (Nonius) markers which are the colored strips on the Mallett test (Figure 2.1). Figure 2.1 shows that there is a great deal of detail surrounding the test to act as a peripheral fusion lock. Also, the letters **O X O** form a central

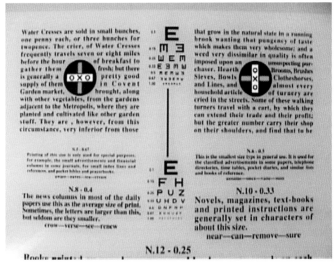

Figure 2.1   Mallett unit fixation disparity test

fusion lock. It is the presence of such a good central and peripheral fusion lock on the Mallett unit that makes this test so valuable. Since the test very closely resembles normal viewing conditions, if a fixation disparity is detected during this test then it is also very likely to be present during everyday life.

Although the Mallett unit test detects fixation disparity, the degree of fixation disparity is not measured with the test. Instead, the test measures the aligning prism (associated heterophoria) or aligning sphere. This is the prism or sphere that is required to align the strips. This is clinically relevant for two reasons:

- the size of the aligning prism (with a genuine Mallett unit) has been correlated with the likelihood of the patient having symptoms
- the aligning prism or sphere is usually equal to the prism or sphere that is required to render the heterophoria compensated.

The exact method and questions that are used with the Mallett unit fixation disparity test have been shown to be important. These are summarized in Table 2.2. All research on this test has used genuine Mallett units. There are some copies which often have differences in design and it is unclear whether these will give the same results.

Using the norms in Table 2.2, the near Mallett unit fixation disparity test has a sensitivity and specificity for detecting symptomatic heterophoria of about 75–80%. For a clinical test, these results are impressive, but are of course not 100%. Therefore other clinical tests are sometimes useful (see Table 2.5) and these will now be described.

Fusional reserves

Figure 1.4 shows that a key factor determining a person's ability to compensate for a heterophoria is the fusional reserve that they use to overcome the heterophoria. This is called the **opposing fusional reserve** and, for example, is the convergent fusional reserve in exophoria. The convergent fusional reserve can be measured by introducing base out prisms. This can be a source of

Table 2.2 Test method and norms for the near Mallett unit fixation disparity test

1. Without the polarized visors, show the patient the horizontal test (green strips vertically placed above and below the **O X O**) and check that the patient perceives both green strips in perfect alignment. Increase ambient illumination
2. Introduce the polarized visor and ask the patient if the two green strips are still **exactly** lined up, whilst they keep their head still
3. If the patient says that they are exactly lined up, then ask if one or both of the strips ever moves a little
4. If (2) or (3) reveals a misalignment, then introduce prisms in front of the relevant eye(s) or spheres in front of both eyes until the strips are aligned and stay aligned. For an exo-slip (right eye's strip moving to the patient's left) add base in prism or minus spheres
5. After changing the prism or spheres, have the patient read a line of text to stabilize their binocular vision before re-testing for fixation disparity
6. Make a note of the results in (4), remove the aligning prism or sphere, and then repeat for the vertical test
7. An aligning prism of 1Δ or more in pre-presbyopes or 2Δ or more in presbyopes is very likely to be associated with symptoms
8. With pre-presbyopes, it is therefore useful to initially introduce prisms in $1/2\Delta$ steps

confusion since when an exophoria is corrected it is bases in prisms that are used. But for fusional reserve testing, the goal is to "create" a larger and larger exophoria to see what the visual system can overcome. So the person is forced to exert their convergent fusional reserves by introducing base out prisms. The method of measurement of fusional reserves is summarized in Table 2.3.

Foveal suppression test

In Chapter 3 sensory adaptations to strabismus are discussed, including patients who develop **global suppression** of the

Table 2.3   Test method and norms for fusional reserves

1.	The most common method is to use a prism bar, but rotary prisms also can be used
2.	Base out prisms are used to measure the convergent fusional reserves, and vice versa
3.	The fusional reserve opposing the heterophoria (convergent in exophoria) should be measured first
4.	Introduce the prism at about the rate of 1Δ per second
5.	The patient should fixate a detailed accommodative target (e.g., vertical line of letters on a budgie stick if testing at near)
6.	First, the patient should report when the target goes blurred, which is recorded as the **blur point**. Sometimes, there is no blur point
7.	The patient should be asked to report when the target goes double: the **break point**. The practitioner should watch the patient's eyes to confirm this objectively
8.	The prism is then reduced until single vision and ocular alignment is restored
9.	Record the results as blur/break/recovery. For example: Fus. Res. N con 12/20/15 div – /10/8 ("–" indicates no blur point)
10.	Results can be compared with norms, but the precise norms depend on the test conditions. It is more meaningful to relate the results to the heterophoria
11.	Sheard's criterion says that the fusional reserve (to blur or if no blur to break) that opposes the heterophoria should be at least twice the heterophoria. For example, if a patient has 8Δ exophoria at near, then their convergent fusional reserve should be at least 16Δ. This criterion works well for exophoria
12.	Percival's criterion says, in essence, that the fusional reserves should be balanced so that the smaller fusional reserve is more than half the larger one. For example, if the convergent fusional reserve to break point is 20Δ, then the divergent fusional reserve should be at least 10Δ. Percival's criterion is useful for esophoric patients

binocular field of the strabismic eye. A rather different form of sensory adaptation can occur in more subtle non-strabismic cases in which a heterophoria is decompensating and yet there are no symptoms. The patient may have poor recovery on cover testing, a fixation disparity that requires a high aligning prism, and fusional reserves that are inadequate for overcoming the heterophoria. Typically, these clinical signs would cause symptoms and yet rare cases are encountered when there are no symptoms, and this can be a puzzling finding. The explanation probably lies in foveal suppression, which can be a sensory adaptation to avoid the symptoms of decompensated heterophoria.

Foveal suppression can prevent symptoms in heterophoria because Panum's fusional areas are smaller at the fovea, so if these are suppressed in one eye then the patient can have a larger fixation disparity without necessarily having any symptoms. Foveal suppression is detected with the foveal suppression test on the Mallett unit (Figure 2.2) and the method of use is described in Table 2.4.

Other tests relevant to the assessment of heterophoria

Only certain key tests for the assessment of heterophoria have been described in this chapter, but many other tests are available that provide additional useful information. Stereo-acuity tests are certainly a useful addition to the routine eye examination: random dot tests are helpful for detecting strabismus, and contoured tests are useful for grading stereo-acuity in heterophoria. The Randot test is particularly useful because it has subtests for both of these types of stereopsis.

Other tests include dissociation tests (e.g., Maddox rod and Maddox wing) and tests of vergence facility and these are described in more detailed texts. Other parts of the routine eye examination provide essential information, such as ophthalmoscopy, pupil reactions, visual fields (when the patient is old enough), refraction, and measurements of accommodative function.

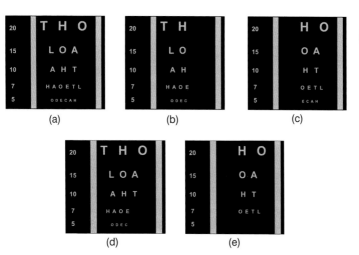

Figure 2.2 Diagram illustrating the use of the Mallett foveal suppression test. The numbers on the left hand side of the test represent the acuity in minutes of arc ('). It is recommended that the patient is only shown the test while wearing the polarized filter, when (depending on the orientation of the polarizers) the right eye sees the image in (b) and the left eye the image in (c). If, for example, a patient reports seeing the letters illustrated in (d), then under binocular conditions the left eye has an acuity if 10' compared with 5' for the right eye. The poorer acuity in the left eye might result from a monocular factor (e.g. refractive error) or a binocular sensory adaptation (e.g. foveal suppression). If, while the polarized filter is still worn, the better eye (right in this example) is covered then the best acuity of the left eye under monocular conditions can be determined. In the example, the patient sees the letters illustrated in (e), so that the patient has foveal suppression of 3' in the left eye (the 10 in (d) less the 7' in (e)) and an acuity of 5' in the right eye and 7' in the left eye (reproduced with permission from Evans, B.J.W. (2002) *Pickwell's Binocular Vision Anomalies*, 4th edition, Butterworth-Heinemann)

Summary of the diagnosis of decompensated heterophoria

To summarize, decompensated heterophoria is diagnosed on the basis of symptoms and the results of a battery of tests. The busy clinician needs to know which tests are most important so that

Table 2.4 Test method and norms for Mallett foveal suppression test

1. It is recommended that the patient is only shown the test (a) whilst wearing the polarized filter, when (depending on the orientation of the polarizers) the right eye sees the image in (b) and the left eye the image in (c)
2. Have the patient hold the test at their normal reading distance, using any glasses that they normally wear for work at that distance
3. Ask the patient to read down the polarized chart, noting how far down they read with each eye
4. If, for example, a patient reports seeing the letters illustrated in (d), then under **binocular viewing conditions** the left eye has an acuity if 10′ compared with 5′ for the right eye. The poorer acuity in the left eye might result from a monocular factor (e.g., refractive error) or a binocular sensory adaptation (e.g., foveal suppression)
5. If, whilst the polarized filter is still worn, the better eye (right in this example) is covered then the best acuity of the left eye under **monocular viewing conditions** can be determined
6. In the example, the patient sees the letters illustrated in (e), so that the patient has foveal suppression of 3′ in the left eye (10′ − 7′)
7. If the best line that the patient can read under binocular conditions (without occlusion) is one line or more worse than under monocular conditions (with occlusion) then this is an abnormal result

they can reach a diagnosis as rapidly and efficiently as possible. Table 2.5 has been reproduced to help with this: it is a simple worksheet which gives an algorithm to assist with the diagnosis of decompensated heterophoria. The last two items in Table 2.5 are designed to detect **binocular instability**, which is a condition related to decompensated heterophoria and which is described on pp. 37–40.

Table 2.5 Scoring system for diagnosing decompensated heterophoria and binocular instability. This scoring algorithm is most appropriate for horizontal heterophoria: for vertical heterophoria, if aligning prism of 0.5Δ or more is detected then, after checking trial frame alignment, measure the vertical dissociated phoria. If this is more than the aligning prism and there are symptoms then diagnose decompensated heterophoria; but still complete the worksheet for any horizontal phoria that may be present

DISTANCE/NEAR (delete)	score
1. Does the patient have one or more of the symptoms of decompensated heterophoria (headache, aching eyes, diplopia, blurred vision difficulty changing focus, distortions, reduced stereopsis, monocular comfort, sore eyes, general irritation)? *If so, score +3 (+2 or +1 if borderline)*	
Are the symptoms at D ☐ or N ☐ *All the following questions apply to D or N, as ticked (if both ticked, complete 2 worksheets)*	
2. Is the patient orthophoric on cover testing? Yes ☐ or No ☐ *If no, score +1*	
3. Is the cover test recovery rapid and smooth? Yes ☐ or No ☐ *If no, score +2 (+1 if borderline)*	
4. Is the Mallett Hz aligning prism: <1Δ for patients under 40, or <2Δ for pxs over 40? Yes ☐ or No ☐ *If no, score +2*	
5. Is the Mallett aligning prism stable (Nonius strips stationary with any required prism)? Yes ☐ or No ☐ *If no, score +1*	
6. Using the polarized letters binocular status test, is any foveal suppression < one line? Yes ☐ or No ☐ *If no, score +2*	
Add up score so far and enter in right hand column	
if score: <4 diagnose normal, >5 treat, 4–5 continue down table adding to score so far	

(continued)

Table 2.5 Continued

DISTANCE/NEAR	(delete)	score
7. Sheard's criterion: (a) measure the dissociated phoria (e.g., Maddox wing, prism cover test); record size & stability (b) measure the fusional reserve opposing the heterophoria (i.e., convergent, or base out, in exophoria). Record as blur/break/recovery in Δ. Is the blur point, or if no blur point the break point, [in (b)] at least twice the phoria [in (a)]? Yes □ or No □		*If no, score +2*
8. Percival's criterion: measure the other fusional reserve and compare the two break points. Is the smaller break point more than half the larger break point? Yes □ or No □		*If no, score +1*
9. When you measured the dissociated heterophoria, was the result stable, or unstable (varying over a range of $\pm 2\Delta$ or more)? (e.g., during Maddox wing test, if the Hz phoria was 4Δ XOP and the arrow was moving from 2 to 6, then result unstable) Stable □ or Unstable □		*If unstable, score +1*
10. Using the fusional reserve measurements, add the divergent break point to the convergent break point. Is the total (=fusional amplitude) at least 20Δ? Yes □ or No □		*If no, score +1*

Add up total score (from both sections of table) and enter in right hand column. If total score: <6 then diagnose compensated heterophoria, if >5 diagnose decompensated heterophoria or binocular instability (see pp. 37–40).

When do I need to do something?

Heterophoria is a normal finding and most cases require no action. Treatment is only required if the heterophoria decompensates. The reasons for this are discussed on pp. 11–12 and illustrated in Figure 1.4.

The general advice on pp. 10–11 about managing binocular vision anomalies apply: action is only required if the binocular vision anomalies are causing problems, are likely to deteriorate if left untreated, or if they are a sign of pathology. It is very rare for decompensated heterophoria to be a sign of ocular pathology, but a marked change in the magnitude of a heterophoria should arouse suspicion. This is one reason why it is useful to always record an estimate of the size of the heterophoria, for example based on cover testing (see Table 1.3).

The investigation of heterophoria is mostly about determining whether it is compensated or not. This was discussed in the previous section.

What do I do?

Decompensated heterophoria is fairly commonly encountered in primary care optometric practice and nearly all cases can be managed in the primary care setting. The main treatment options are listed below:

1. remove the cause of decompensation
2. eye exercises
3. refractive modification
4. prismatic correction
5. surgery.

The required treatment will depend on the conditions of the particular case. This will partly depend on the type of heterophoria (discussed on pp. 2–3), but will also depend on patient characteristics (e.g., age, motivation, etc.). These factors now will be considered as the treatment options outlined above are considered in turn.

1. Remove the cause of decompensation

A consideration of Figure 1.4 will reveal the main factors that can cause decompensation. For example, if working under dim lighting is causing poor sensory fusion then the appropriate treatment is to increase the lighting. If anisometropia or cataract is causing poor sensory fusion then appropriate treatments are contact lenses and surgery, respectively. Correcting refractive errors, even sometimes if they are quite small, can aid sensory fusion.

Monovision can be a successful method of correcting presbyopia either with contact lenses or refractive surgery. But monovision could also be described as induced anisometropia, and it is therefore contraindicated in people who have a heterophoria which is not well-compensated.

2. Eye exercises

Eye exercises are most likely to be effective in small or moderate exophoria. It is harder to achieve success with exercises for esophoria and much harder (arguably impossible) for hyperphoria. Exercises can work in patients of any age, but the patient needs to be old enough to understand what is required and in older people the exercises tend to take longer to work. Without doubt, the most important factor is patient motivation: if the patient lacks motivation and enthusiasm then exercises are very unlikely to be effective.

The purpose of eye exercises for decompensated heterophoria is to increase the fusional reserve that opposes the heterophoria; for example, to increase the convergent fusional reserves in exophoria. Exophoric conditions are treated most often in this way and will be described here. Similar principles apply to the training of divergent fusional reserves in esophoria.

Controlled trials show that convergent fusional reserves can be trained with exercises, and a key component is probably the mental effort to keep the eyes over-converged during the exercises. Exercises may use a haploscopic device (e.g., a form of stereoscope) or free-space techniques. Free-space techniques are probably the most common form of fusional reserve exercises these days, and can be further sub-divided into two types:

- exercises where convergence and accommodation are kept associated in the usual way and are trained together. These exercises are most commonly used when there is a convergence insufficiency as part of the problem and are described on pp. 37–39.

- Exercises where the link between convergence and accommodation is dissociated. The best known of these is probably the **three cats exercise**, described in Figure 2.3 and Table 2.6.

A problem with the three cats exercise, or similar approaches, is that patients rapidly become bored. This led to the development at the Institute of Optometry of the Institute Free-space Stereogram (IFS) exercises (Figure 2.4), the features of which are described in Table 2.7. The idea behind the IFS exercises is that the parent (or for older patients, the patient themselves) becomes the vision therapist. There are very detailed instructions that the parent reads out to the child whilst the child views a series of targets on cards. Each card is different, with a variety of tasks for the patient to do, which prevents boredom. The child perceives a marked '3-D' effect, which also helps maintain interest. There are a series of self-checks where the parent asks

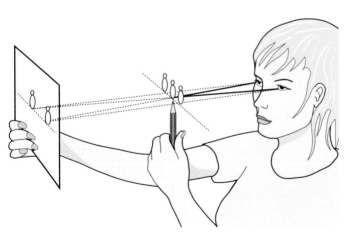

Figure 2.3 'Three cats' exercise. See Table 2.6.
(Reproduced with permission from Evans, B.J.W. (1997), *Pickwell's Binocular Vision Anomalies*, 3rd edition, Butterworth-Heinemann)

Table 2.6 **Method of use of the 'three cats' exercise**

1.	The card with drawings of two incomplete cats is held at arm's length
2.	The patient fixates on a pencil held between the card and the eyes
3.	Physiological diplopic images of the cats will be seen as blurred images, and the pencil distance adjusted until the middle two cats fuse into a complete cat with two incomplete cats, one each side (the resultant percept is of three cats)
4.	The patient is asked to try to see the cats clearly. This involves maintaining convergence for the pencil distance and relaxing accommodation (exercising negative relative accommodation)
5.	Typically, the exercise is carried out for 10 minutes twice a day
6.	The patient should be checked again soon, typically after about 3 weeks

Table 2.7 **Goals and design features of IFS exercises**

Goal	Design feature
Affordable	Printed home exercises
Easy to understand	Comprehensive instructions
Fun to do	Novel 3-D images Varied tasks
Motivating	Encourage parent/child team One or two 10 min sessions daily Check in 3–4 weeks
Checks on progress	10 self-test questions
Variety of stimuli	18 targets with step and ramp Different size stimuli Different shape stimuli Vergence angles: 3–30Δ
Control/treat suppression	Physiological diplopic images Monocular markers Stereopsis

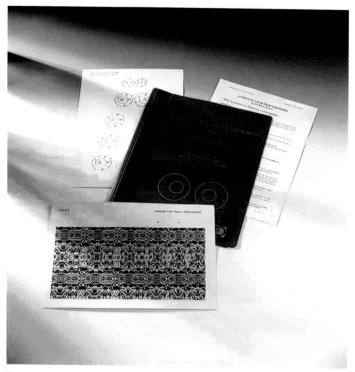

Figure 2.4 Institute Free-space Stereogram (IFS) exercises. Reproduced with permission of i.O.O. Sales (www.ioosales.co.uk)

the child a question to check if they are doing the exercises properly. If not, then the parent is instructed to contact the practitioner (this only rarely occurs).

The IFS exercises include four cards for the patient to view, some of which have ring targets with objects that are seen in depth and others with autostereograms (e.g., in the foreground of Figure 2.4). The autostereograms have been designed so that, if the patient is over-converging appropriately, they see a series of steps which appear to 'come off the page' towards them. Each time they have the perception of moving up a step their eyes have to over-converge to a greater degree. On each step is a letter and if the child identifies the letter correctly then the parent knows that they are doing the exercises properly. These exercises have proved popular with both optometrists and orthoptists.

It should be stressed that there are literally dozens of different types of fusional reserve exercises and only a brief introduction has been given here. The IFS exercises are suitable for use by the patient at home. This is a popular approach with many practitioners, although some practitioners prefer treatment in the practice. The more complex cases may require a battery of exercises rather than just one type. A key factor is the ability of the patient and (if a child) their parent to understand the instructions and the practitioner must check that these are fully understood before the patient leaves the practice. It is generally advisable to give written instructions, like those that are included with the IFS exercises.

Most practitioners would agree that it is much better to have a brief period of "aggressive" exercises (e.g., 2–3 times a day for 10–15 minutes a time for 3 weeks) rather than a half-hearted attempt to do the exercises over several months. Ideally a follow-up appointment should be booked about 3 weeks after the exercises are issued. Another advantage of this approach is that, if the exercises are not working, this fact is identified rapidly so that another management option (or referral) can be pursued.

3. Refractive modification

In some cases an uncorrected refractive error is the cause for the decompensated heterophoria. For example, there may be uncorrected hypermetropia in esophoria, uncorrected myopia in exophoria, or astigmatism impairing sensory fusion. In these cases, the refractive correction is the only proper treatment, since this will remove the cause of decompensation.

In other cases there may be no significant refractive error, or a refractive error that is already being adequately corrected, and yet a **refractive modification** might be an appropriate method of correcting the decompensated heterophoria. A common use of this approach is in patients with convergence excess esophoria: an esophoria that is worse at near than at distance. Bifocal or varifocal spectacles would be likely to render the heterophoria compensated.

Many decompensated exophorias are also very amenable to treatment in this way. A **"negative add"** can be used (e.g., giving minus lenses to an emmetrope) to induce accommodative convergence which helps the patient to overcome an exophoria. It is important to explain to the patient and the parent that these are **exercise glasses** and the goal is to reduce the "add" over time as the patient gradually becomes able, by increasing degrees, to compensate for the deviation. This very simple method of treatment is often highly effective and is sadly under-used. The method is summarized in Table 2.8.

The patients who are most amenable to treatment by refractive modification are those with a high AC/A ratio. The AC/A ratio defines how much the vergence changes per diopter of accommodation. For example, during a Maddox Wing test a patient might have an esophoria of 8Δ. If +2.00DS lenses are added, the esophoria reduces to 2Δ. The vergence has changed by 6Δ (8–2) for 2D of relaxation in accommodation, so the AC/A ratio is $3\Delta/D$ (6/2). A value of $3–4\Delta/D$ is normal.

4. Prismatic correction

Prismatic correction is quite commonly used to correct a decompensated heterophoria in older patients, typically as base in prism in reading glasses. Small vertical heterophoria, although rare, also responds well to prisms. In other cases prisms may be used as a temporary correction, for example in a child who is taking examinations and who will return for exercises in the school holidays. The method is summarized in Table 2.9.

5. Surgery

Surgery is only very rarely required for decompensated heterophoria. Typically, these are the cases where the heterophoria is very large and is causing considerable symptoms, yet is too large to treat with the other methods described above. These cases will require referral to a surgeon.

Table 2.8 **Method of use for refractive modification to treat decompensated heterophoria**

1. Using the Mallett fixation disparity unit (see Table 2.2) at the appropriate distance investigate the minimum refractive modification that is required to bring the polarized strips into alignment. For example, in exophoria increase the minus until the strips are aligned

2. Remove the polarized visor and check the visual acuities at the appropriate distance. In the case of a negative add, this checks that the accommodation is adequately overcoming the minus: this method of treatment is only appropriate in patients with adequate accommodation

3. Have the patient read a couple of lines of text through the lenses to stabilize their binocular vision. Then check the cover test to make sure that the heterophoria appears reasonably well-compensated (see Table 1.4)

4. Advise the spectacles to be worn for concentrated visual tasks at the appropriate distance or, if symptoms or the risk of strabismus are severe, all the time

5. Prescribe the spectacles (or contact lenses), annotating the prescription to state 'Refractive modification to treat decompensated heterophoria'. Explain this to the patient and parent/carer

6. Advise the patient to return immediately if they have any diplopia or any persistent blurred vision or asthenopia

7. Check again in 3 months, repeating steps 1–5 and reducing the refractive modification when you can

Table 2.9   Method of use of prismatic correction for decompensated heterophoria

1. Using the Mallett fixation disparity unit (see Table 2.2) at the appropriate distance, investigate the minimum prismatic correction modification that is required to bring the polarized strips into alignment. For example, in exophoria increase the base in until the strips are aligned

2. Have the patient read a couple of lines of text through the lenses to stabilize their binocular vision. Then check the cover test to make sure that the heterophoria appears reasonably well-compensated (see Table 1.4)

3. Patients with abnormal binocular vision usually do not adapt to prisms, but this can be checked by repeating steps 1–2 after the patient has read for about 3 minutes

Specific types of heterophoria

Mixed esophoria (basic esophoria)

In mixed esophoria the esophoria is similar at distance and near. If it is decompensated then it may need treatment at both distances. A cycloplegic refraction is mandatory in these cases and if significant hypermetropia is found or if the patient is decompensated then plus should be prescribed. These cases need to be monitored frequently since sometimes they can decompensate (even if fully corrected), for example during febrile illnesses. Parents need to be taught to look for a turning eye and advised to seek professional care if this occurs at any time.

   If an esophoria is decompensating, but not at a specific distance, and is not fully accommodative (not fully corrected by the maximum plus revealed by cycloplegia) then management options (in addition to maximum plus) are eye exercises, prisms or surgery.

Divergence weakness (distance esophoria)

In divergence weakness the esophoria is significantly greater at distance and, as in any case of significant esophoria, a cycloplegic refraction is usually indicated. It is also important to rule out the possibility of a lateral rectus palsy (see Table 6.9). Decompensated divergence weakness esophoria is uncommon and is often very difficult to treat in primary eyecare practices. Occasionally, they may respond to exercises to increase the divergent fusional reserves at distance. Suitable methods are beyond the scope of this book (see *Pickwell's Binocular Vision Anomalies* for further explanation).

Convergence excess (near esophoria)

In these cases the esophoria is significantly greater at near. Once latent hypermetropia has been ruled out, then multifocals are often the most appropriate management (see pp. 32–33).

Mixed exophoria (basic exophoria)

In mixed exophoria the exophoria is similar at distance and near. If these cases decompensate, then eye exercises or a negative add are often successful treatments.

Divergence excess (distance exophoria)

In divergence excess exophoria there is an exophoria which is significantly greater at distance than at near. Many of these cases are really intermittent exotropia since friends and family notice a large divergent deviation when the patient looks into the far distance, of which the patient is usually unaware because they suppress. To the practitioner, who works at a maximum distance of 6 m, these cases usually appear as a distance exophoria and they will therefore be discussed in this section.

Some of these cases respond to exercises to increase the convergent fusional reserves. For example, they can be loaned a prism bar and taught to look at a distant object and to try and

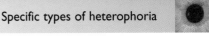

maintain fusion as the base out prism is increased. Cases where the patient is completely unaware when an eye drifts out can be very difficult to treat because they suppress during exercises. For these cases, orthoptic exercises are much easier with haploscopic devices.

Some of these cases can be treated successfully with a "negative add", and the technique for this is described in Table 2.8. The Mallett unit fixation disparity test can be used to check whether this would give the patient an unacceptable esophoria at near. If this is a concern, then multifocals can be prescribed.

Convergence weakness (near exophoria)

In convergence weakness exophoria, the exophoria is significantly greater at near than at distance. If the near exophoria is decompensated then it can be treated as outlined on pp. 28–34. Eye exercises usually work well for these cases. Convergence weakness exophoria is often (but not always) associated with convergence insufficiency (see below), and when it is then treatment of the convergence insufficiency often improves the person's ability to compensate for the exophoria.

Convergence insufficiency

Convergence insufficiency is characterized by a remote near point of convergence: usually it is more remote than 8–10 cm. This condition is often (but not always) associated with convergence weakness exophoria. Convergence insufficiency is very amenable to treatment with eye exercises, and examples, in increasing order of complexity, are listed in Table 2.10. Table 2.10 stresses the need to keep the object single, but usually the patient is asked to also keep the object clear. This is especially important where the patient has a combined convergence and accommodative insufficiency (see Chapter 8). In older patients, where the near point of accommodation may naturally be further out than the near point of convergence, then the instructions should stress single vision (as in Table 2.10), not clear vision, and non-accommodative targets will be more appropriate.

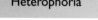

Table 2.10 Examples of eye exercises for convergence insufficiency

Type of exercise	Details of exercise
Simple push-up	1. The patient views a detailed near target and brings it towards their nose, trying to keep it single for as long as possible 2. When the target doubles, they move back out and repeat stage 1
Push-up with physiological diplopia	1. As above, but the patient also holds a second target a few centimeters beyond the first 2. The distal target is seen in physiological diplopia and the patient is made aware of this 3. They must keep fixating the nearer target, but keep aware of the furthest which must be seen in physiological diplopia all the time 4. If physiological diplopia is lost, then move the targets out until it is regained. In other respects, the exercise is carried out as for the **simple push-up** method
Distance to near (jump convergence)	1. The patient views a detailed near target and brings it towards their nose, trying to keep it single for as long as possible. The distance when doubling occurs is the near point of convergence 2. This **near target** is then held just beyond this point 3. The patient then looks at a distant target and makes this single 4. Then the patient looks back at the near target, making this single 5. Steps 3 and 4 are repeated, every now and then checking that the near target is close to the near point of convergence
Distance to near (jump convergence) with physiological diplopia	1. As above, but the patient holds an additional target a few centimeters beyond the near target 2. This target is seen in physiological diplopia and the patient is made aware of this

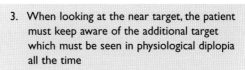
	3. When looking at the near target, the patient must keep aware of the additional target which must be seen in physiological diplopia all the time
Bead-on-string	1. This approach is particularly suitable for patients with quite marked convergence insufficiency (e.g., NPC 20 cm or greater)
	2. A bead (or nut) is threaded onto a piece of string. The patient holds the piece of string on the bridge of their nose, with the other end held at arm's length or tied to an object directly in front of the patient
	3. The bead is placed further away from the patient than the near point of convergence and the patient should see a single bead. The string should form an X, centered on the bead. This needs to be pointed out to the patient as this awareness of physiological diplopia can be used to check for suppression
	4. The bead is gradually moved towards the patient until diplopia (or suppression)
	5. The same method of "pushing up" to the patient is used as in the first two methods described above, but also maintaining an awareness of the string forming an X

Binocular instability

The eyeballs are visco-elastic spheres surrounded by relatively soft orbital fat and connective tissue. Considering this, and the fact that the eyes move at incredibly high speeds, it is amazing that they usually keep as well co-ordinated as they do. It is not surprising that small vergence errors occur, and it was noted above that Panum's fusional areas allow some "free play" in the sensory visual system. Similarly, the fusional reserves allow some tolerance in the motor system. This is why orthophoric patients still need to possess fusional reserves. A corollary of this is that patients with very low fusional reserves or with impaired sensory fusion might, even if they have orthophoria or minimal heterophoria, still have trouble maintaining fusion and may consequently have symptoms (Figure 1.4). This condition is called **binocular instability**.

A patient with binocular instability might have the symptoms of decompensated heterophoria and yet only have a negligible heterophoria. But the fusional reserves will be very low and/or there will be an impairment to sensory fusion (e.g., anisometropia).

The fusional reserves tend to be, on average, lower in people who are dyslexic than in good readers. So, people with dyslexia (or specific learning difficulties) are a little more likely than usual to have binocular instability. To test for this, it is important to ask if there is any movement of the Nonius markers in the Mallett fixation disparity test and to measure the fusional reserves. In binocular instability there is usually excessive movement of the Nonius markers, excessive movement of the arrow in the Maddox wing test, and a low fusional amplitude. In Table 2.5, items 5, 9 and 10 refer to binocular instability.

3
Strabismus

What is strabismus?

Strabismus occurs when the visual axes are misaligned: the two eyes do not point directly at the object of regard. Panum's fusional area allows some free play in the visual system: the visual axes can be slightly misaligned (by a few minutes of arc; fixation disparity) without the patient losing normal binocular vision. Strabismus usually signifies a deviation that is an order of magnitude greater than this: typically, the visual axes are misaligned by several degrees, rather than minutes of arc. An exception to this is microtropia, when the visual axes are misaligned by less than 10Δ; this is discussed in Chapter 4. When the visual axes are misaligned by an amount that is too great to allow sensory fusion within Panum's fusional areas then a strabismus is present. Small angle strabismus may not be recognizable by looking at the patient and it is these cases that are particularly challenging for the eyecare professional to determine.

Sensory adaptations to strabismus

Strabismic amblyopia is a sensory consequence of strabismus and is discussed in Chapter 5. The present chapter covers sensory adaptations to strabismus, which can be thought of as diplopia-avoiding mechanisms. In strabismus, since the visual axes point at different objects the patient might be expected to have diplopia, and if they are too old to develop sensory adaptations then this is what will happen. To avoid diplopia, younger patients with strabismus must either suppress the entire binocular field of their strabismic eye or develop harmonious anomalous retinal correspondence (HARC). HARC can be thought of as a "re-wiring" of retinal correspondence so that the patient has a form of pseudo-correspondence. HARC works especially well in microtropia, and is discussed in this context in Chapter 4.

The other sensory adaptation to avoid diplopia in strabismus is suppression. In Chapter 2 we discussed foveal suppression, which is most likely to occur in decompensated heterophoria. The suppression that occurs to avoid diplopia in strabismus is rather different since the whole binocular field of the strabismic eye will need to be suppressed. For this reason, the suppression in strabismus has been called **global suppression**.

Rather confusingly, patients who, instead of global suppression have HARC, often have two small suppression areas in their strabismic eye's visual field: one at the fovea of their strabismic eye and one at the zero point. The zero point is the part of the strabismic eye's visual field that neo-corresponds with the fovea of the non-strabismic eye. The reason that these two small suppression areas are necessary is because it is at the two foveae that Panum's fusional areas are very small, and this makes anomalous correspondence at these two positions very difficult. It should be stressed that these two small suppression areas occur in the presence of HARC, and are quite different to the global suppression which occurs as the alternative diplopia avoidance mechanism to HARC. For this reason, these small suppression areas have been called **local suppression areas**. These local suppression areas in HARC have been said to subtend 1–2°, although it is sometimes argued that they are in some cases larger and can coalesce into one suppression area, with HARC existing in the periphery. The debate over this is probably fuelled by the fact that the dimensions of these areas may not be fixed, but may vary with different test conditions.

The factors that predispose a patient to develop either HARC or global suppression are summarized in Table 3.1. It should be

Table 3.1 **Factors which influence the likelihood of a child with strabismus developing either HARC or global suppression. Note: exceptions to these tendencies occur in some cases**

Factor	More likely to develop HARC	More likely to develop global suppression
Size of deviation	Small	Large
Stability of deviation	Constant	Variable
Type of deviation	Esotropia	Exotropia
Age of onset	Young child	Older child

noted that the table only represents tendencies: there are many exceptions who have not followed the predispositions in Table 3.1. A useful mnemonic is that the factors favoring HARC can be remembered as the five S's: **s**mall, **s**table, e**s**o, **s**tarted **s**oon.

How do I investigate?

As in any binocular vision anomalies, it is important to be sure of the nature of the condition. For example, regular checks on ocular health and comitancy should take place. Indeed, all the factors in Table 3.3 need to be regularly reviewed.

Motor

It is important to know the size of the deviation, since any change in the angle must be detectable. But it must be borne in mind that this is likely to increase with increasing degrees of dissociation. The standard method is the cover test (see Figure 1.2 and Table 1.1), recording the size of deviation (Table 1.3) on the initial covering and then the degree to which this "builds" with repeat covering (Table 1.5).

Other dissociation tests can also be used to obtain an estimate of the degree of deviation, such as a Maddox wing or Maddox rod. If deep sensory adaptations are present then these can interfere with the measurement, and some alternating covering may be necessary to break down the adaptation, but this will be likely to increase the angle.

Sensory

HARC is an acquired adaptation and it must be remembered that normal retinal correspondence is still the innate correspondence which will be present "underneath" the adaptation. If the patient is presented with artificial test situations then the adaptation can be "broken down" and the patient may revert to normal retinal correspondence. Of course, they will still have the strabismus so if they revert to normal retinal correspondence then they will have diplopia at this point in the test. The goal of clinical tests is to determine the sensory adaptations that operate during the patient's normal everyday visual activities. To do this, the clinical tests need to replicate these everyday conditions as accurately as possible: they should be naturalistic. This is why artificial, dissociating, instruments such as a synoptophore are inappropriate for determining sensory status. The two best tests are the Bagolini Lens Test and the Mallett Modified OXO Test (Figure 3.1). Nearly all primary eyecare practices have a Mallett unit, so this technique will be described here.

The small OXO tests, which are designed to detect fixation disparity in the presence of heterophoria, should not be used to test for HARC or global suppression. This is because of the small local suppression areas that can occur in HARC (see p. 43) and which can cause the Nonius strip with the small OXO tests to disappear which could cause HARC to be mis-diagnosed as global

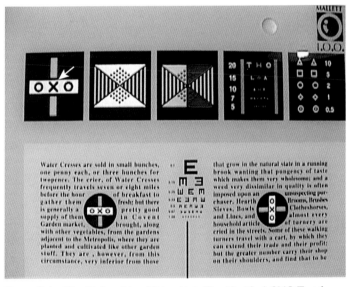

Figure 3.1   The Mallett Near Vision Unit. The Modified OXO Test for testing for HARC or global suppression is the top left large OXO test (courtesy of i.O.O. Sales Ltd.)

suppression. This is why modern versions of the near Mallett unit have the large OXO test (top left hand test in Figure 3.1), best described as the Modified OXO Test for HARC/global suppression. For distance vision testing, the distance OXO fixation disparity test can be used at the modified testing distance of 1.5 m: at this distance the larger angle that the test subtends makes it suitable.

The method of use of the test is to insert the polarized visor over any refractive correction that the patient usually wears at that distance and, as with any polarized test, to increase the ambient illumination to counteract the light-absorbing effect of the polarized filters. The patient is directed to look at the large modified OXO and to describe what they see, whilst they look at the X. If they have normal retinal correspondence then they should experience diplopia, as in the third panel on the bottom row of Figure 3.2. If they see only one green strip, which should correspond to the non-strabismic eye (second panel bottom row of Figure 3.2), then they have global suppression of their strabismic eye. If a strabismic patient sees both green strips simultaneously but only one OXO then they must have HARC

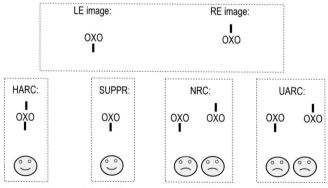

Modified OXO test

Figure 3.2 Use of the Mallett Modified OXO Test to detect HARC or global suppression in strabismus (reproduced with permission from *Optician*, 11 June, 1999, No. 5705, Vol. 217)

(first panel bottom row of Figure 3.2). It is unlikely that the anomalous correspondence will create the perfect perception of normal binocular vision: it is quite likely that the Nonius strip in the strabismic eye will be a different size or brightness to the strip from the other eye or it may even flicker. These reports do not normally indicate any significant problems.

During the test for HARC or suppression it is advisable to check the motor status by carrying out a cover test. This should confirm that the strabismus is still present and that the patient has not changed fixation to the other eye.

Some patients have very deep sensory adaptations, whereas in other cases the sensory adaptations are quite lightly ingrained. Patients with deep sensory adaptations are likely to exhibit the characteristics favoring the development of HARC in the first place (see Table 3.1) and are unlikely to require treatment of their strabismus, or indeed to be amenable to treatment of this. The depth of the sensory adaptation can be measured by observing how easily their sensory adaptation is embarrassed. The most common method is to introduce a neutral density filter bar between the polarized visor and the eye. If the patient has HARC then the filter bar is introduced in front of the strabismic eye until the HARC breaks down. If they have global suppression then the filter bar is introduced in front of the dominant eye until the suppression of the other eye breaks down.

This section has described the three most common forms of sensory status in strabismus: HARC, global suppression, or normal retinal correspondence with diplopia. A fourth option, unharmonious retinal correspondence (Figure 3.1), is hardly ever encountered in primary eyecare practice. For a description of this the reader should consult a more detailed text.

When do I need to do something?

Table 1.7 listed the three reasons why binocular vision anomalies may require an intervention. Each of these three reasons will now be considered in turn, with respect to strabismus.

1. If the strabismus is causing symptoms or decreased visual function

When young children (below the age of 8–11 years) develop strabismus then they usually acquire sensory adaptations to avoid diplopia (see pp. 42–44). Patients who are too old to develop these adaptations typically experience diplopia in response to a new strabismus. Clearly, these patients will require an intervention, and most cases that are detected in community eyecare practices will require referral to investigate the cause of the strabismus.

Most cases with long-standing small angle strabismus have deeply ingrained sensory adaptations (e.g., HARC; see pp. 42–44) and are asymptomatic. Rarely, cases are encountered where the adaptations to strabismus break down and the patient experiences symptoms. Treating these cases is only appropriate for practitioners with specialist knowledge of binocular vision anomalies and is beyond the scope of this book. A priority is to determine the reason for the patient's sensory adaptations breaking down: if the angle of the strabismus has changed then this will need investigation (see Table 3.3).

If a patient has a large angle strabismus then they may need an intervention for cosmetic reasons. These cases are most likely to require surgery.

The issue of whether a strabismus is causing decreased visual function to a degree that requires treatment is contentious. First, it should be noted that any amblyopia will need treatment as outlined in Chapter 5: in this section we are concentrating on binocular factors. If the strabismus is of small angle (cosmetically good) and there are good sensory adaptations then one school of thought is that the strabismus is unlikely to need treatment and is best left alone. Indeed, to attempt treatment of the motor deviation might interfere with the sensory adaptations and could cause intractable diplopia. Another school of thought is that a patient with strabismus never achieves the binocularity of a patient with true binocular vision, so if the angle can be easily straightened then this should be attempted. Some practitioners argue that the angle and any binocular sensory adaptations should be treated aggressively, with the goal of restoring the best possible binocular vision. In reality, very few practitioners would recommend surgery for a cosmetically good small angle strabismus and there are not many practitioners who would recommend eye exercises for this type of case either. If a patient is very committed (e.g., to meet vocational requirements), then eye exercises aimed at (a) increasing the fusional reserves and (b) eliminating the sensory adaptation are a possibility. Again, there is a risk of producing intractable diplopia so treatment of these cases should only be attempted by appropriately experienced practitioners with the full informed consent of the patient.

If surgery and eye exercises are unlikely treatments for patients with adapted small angle strabismus, then the only treatments for the angle that are left to consider are refractive or prismatic approaches. The most likely of these two to be encountered is refractive treatment. The case example in Table 3.2 illustrates a scenario that might be encountered. Although the child in Table 3.2 is asymptomatic, the hypermetropia is likely to produce symptoms at some stage when it will require correction. To correct this now would be expected to reduce the angle of strabismus. Indeed, if the child has a normal AC/A ratio (e.g., 4Δ/D; see p. 33) then full refractive correction might be expected to eliminate the deviation. In this type of case the sensory adaptation (typically, HARC) usually

Table 3.2 **Case example of uncorrected hypermetrope with esotropia. The management is discussed in the text**

BACKGROUND: Boy, aged 6, first eye examination (no glasses)	
SYMPTOMS: None. Family history of hypermetropia	
CLINICAL FINDINGS: Normal: ocular health, visual acuities, visual fields, ocular motility	
Refractive error:	R=L=+2.50DS
Cycloplegic:	R=L=+3.25DS
Cover test:	D=N=12Δ LSOT
Modified OXO test:	HARC
Stereopsis (Randot):	no random dot or contoured stereopsis

seems to revert back to normal retinal correspondence when the angle is corrected, suggesting that the sensory adaptation is only lightly ingrained. Indeed, since the hypermetropia is likely to need correction at some stage, then it is advisable to correct this as young as possible, since any sensory adaptation is only likely to become more deeply ingrained with age. It is easy to confirm that a refractive correction is safe: simply put the proposed correction in a trial frame and check that the child does not experience diplopia. At the same time, the effect of the correction on the deviation can be checked with a cover test. Before dispensing, explain to the parent that if there are any reports of diplopia then spectacle wear should be ceased and a re-examination booked as soon as possible.

2. If the situation is likely to worsen if left untreated

This is particularly relevant for intermittent strabismus, which can sometimes be an intermediate stage in the development of a constant strabismus. If a practitioner sees a child with an intermittent strabismus then an intervention is necessary because it is much easier to correct an intermittent strabismus than a constant strabismus. This is particularly true of a hypermetropic patient whose esophoria is breaking down into an esotropia. If the hypermetropia is the cause of the esotropia then correcting the hypermetropia will cure the deviation and the appropriate prescription should be prescribed without delay.

Another way in which the situation can worsen if left untreated is with strabismic amblyopia. It is generally thought that it is best to treat this as young as possible, although it probably remains treatable until the age of 7–12 years. Certainly, strabismic amblyopia below the age of 8 years should be treated as soon as it is diagnosed, and this is discussed in Chapter 5.

3. If the strabismus is likely to be a sign of ophthalmic or systemic pathology

Practitioners need to take several steps to determine whether strabismus is likely to result from ocular or systemic pathology. These are summarized in Table 3.3. It is widely accepted that new

Table 3.3 Summary of steps in determining if pathology is present in strabismus

Step	Rationale	What to do
Detect incomitancy	Any new or changing incomitancy requires prompt referral to a hospital ophthalmological unit	• Carry out a careful motility test, including questions about diplopia • If the results are unclear, then carry out a cover test in peripheral gaze or ideally a Hess screen test • If there is a new or changing incomitancy then refer
Look for orbital pathology	Orbital pathology can cause strabismus, although this is rare	• Is proptosis present? • Are the eye movements restricted? • Is there pain on eye movements?
Detect any ocular pathology	Pathology that destroys or diminishes the vision in a significant part of the visual field of one eye can dissociate the eyes and cause strabismus	• Check pupil reactions, particularly looking for an APD • Carry out careful ophthalmoscopy. In younger children, dilated fundoscopy might be necessary to obtain a good view, commonly after cycloplegic refraction. Keep checking ophthalmoscopy at regular intervals • As soon as the child is old enough, check visual fields
Look for neurological problems	Pathology in the brain can cause comitant as well as incomitant deviations	• Carefully check pupil reactions • Assess and record optic disc appearance in both eyes, ideally with photographs • Monitor reports of general health (see text)

(Continued)

Table 3.3 **Continued**

Step	Rationale	What to do
Look for obvious causes of the strabismus	There will be a reason why a patient develops a strabismus. If you find a non-pathological reason, then the likelihood of there being a pathological reason is greatly reduced	• E.g., if a child has an esotropia, then look for latent hypermetropia • E.g., if an older patient is developing an exotropia, then have they always had an exophoria which is gradually decompensating with worsening cataract • In every case, still look for pathology. But if you have found an obvious cause, then it is probably **the** cause
Monitor the size of the deviation	If the deviation is increasing then there must be a reason	• If you cannot find the reason why a deviation is increasing, then refer so that someone else can give a second opinion
Is the strabismus responding to treatment?	If you think that you are treating the cause of the strabismus (e.g., hypermetropia) then the situation should improve	• If a strabismus does not respond to treatment (e.g., giving post-cyclopegic plus for hypermetropia) then review your diagnosis (e.g., accommodative esotropia) • Failure to respond to treatment might indicate a pathological cause, so refer for a second opinion

cases of strabismus do not routinely require brain scans, unless suspicious signs are detected. Whether these cases are seen in primary or secondary care, they need the same initial investigations. Careful checks of ocular health (see Table 3.3), binocular status, and refraction are required. The refraction will detect the cause in many cases, and in others the assessment of binocular status will identify the cause. Less commonly ocular pathology will be present and might be detected with the ophthalmoscope. If an obvious cause of the strabismus is found (e.g., hypermetropia in accommodative esotropia), then this is treated. In these cases, the patient only requires further investigation if the findings are suspicious, or if the situation worsens or does not respond to treatment (see Table 3.3). It is important to monitor the general health of the patient. If this is poor or there are other signs that are suggestive of neurological problems (e.g., headaches, tremor, unusual gait) then this raises the index of suspicion and referral is indicated.

What do I do?

Intermittent strabismus can be thought of as one step worse than decompensated heterophoria, and the same considerations apply as for treating decompensated heterophoria (pp. 27–35). Since the strabismus is intermittent, the patient is likely to have normal retinal correspondence and binocular single vision when the strabismus is not present. So, if the deviation is treated by any of the methods on pp. 27–35 then sensory factors are unlikely to cause problems.

If children with strabismus are seen within the sensitive period (until the age of 7–12 years) then treatment of any amblyopia is a priority. This is discussed in Chapter 5.

New or changed strabismus

Sometimes, the history or symptoms indicate that a strabismus is of recent onset and in these cases it is essential that the practitioner (a) tries to find the cause of the strabismus and refers if they cannot find the cause and (b) treats the strabismus or refers to another practitioner for treatment. Strabismus can be subdivided into various types and the relevant investigative and treatment approaches are analogous to those for the equivalent forms of heterophoria (pp. 34–37).

As always, practitioners need to be alert to the risk of a pathological cause for the deviation. Table 3.3 lists some of the features that help to determine whether pathology is present. Clearly, if there is a significant risk of pathology being present then the patient will require referral to a hospital eye department for investigation.

The cases that are most amenable to treatment in a primary care setting are those in which a comitant deviation of recent onset is found which is clearly of refractive origin. Most commonly, these will be eso-deviations with uncorrected hypermetropia. If correction of the hypermetropia straightens the deviation then the cause of the deviation and the only correct treatment for the deviation have been found. Occasionally, cases are seen in which the development of myopia has caused an exophoria to decompensate and break down into an exotropia. The visual axes can sometimes be straightened by correcting the myopia. In these simple cases where appropriate refractive correction straightens the visual axes then any amblyopia may resolve without treatment, or may require patching (see Chapter 5). The patient should be monitored closely, even if no amblyopia is present, to confirm the diagnosis of purely refractive strabismus. If the strabismus is corrected with the refractive correction and any heterophoria is stable and there are no other risk factors (see Table 3.3) then these cases would not require referral.

In cases where there is not a simple refractive etiology for the strabismus then the index of suspicion for pathology is raised and most of these cases seen in primary eyecare practices will require referral (Table 3.3). An exception might be, for example, if a practitioner has been monitoring a long-standing just compensated heterophoria which, following an event which compromises the compensation, breaks down into a strabismus of similar angle to the original heterophoria. For example, a febrile illness or development of anisometropia might cause the motor or sensory fusion to break down (see Figure 1.4). If an optometrist can treat these cases and restore fusion then they might not require referral, as long as other risk factors are not identified (see Table 3.3). The patient is particularly likely to respond to treatment if they are seen soon after the decompensation occurs, and treatments outlined on pp. 27–37 for decompensated heterophoria should be considered.

Long-standing strabismus

Approximately 2–4% of the population have a strabismus, so primary eyecare practitioners will often encounter patients attending for routine eye examinations who have a long-standing strabismus. Typically these cases will be adults: if previously untreated strabismic amblyopia is detected in children who are at the upper age range for patching (7–12 years) then urgent treatment is required by a practitioner who is able to monitor treatment carefully to ensure that any binocular sensory adaptation is not adversely affected by patching (Chapter 5).

In most cases of adults with long-standing strabismus, the patient will report a history of a long-standing deviation that is not changing and they will have no symptoms relating to their strabismus. The usual advice for such cases is that if the strabismus is not causing any problems then it does not require any treatment. Indeed, if there is any pre-existing prismatic correction, spectacle lens decentration, or partial correction of anisometropia then it is best to mimic this in any new refractive correction.

Comitant (or indeed incomitant) strabismus can decompensate and worsen at any time in life. This is one reason why it is useful to measure the angle in these cases so that any change can be detected in the future, although this is usually obvious from the patient's symptoms. A strabismus that is changing will require referral to find the reason why it is changing (see Table 3.3). This may be idiopathic, but should still be investigated and may require surgery. One possible reason why a long-standing unilateral strabismus with sensory adaptation might break down is if the patient's sensory status is changed. This might occur, for example, if the patient is prescribed monovision contact lenses or monovision refractive surgery. Monovision is therefore contraindicated in these cases.

Occasionally, patients will be encountered who have a stable long-standing strabismus that is cosmetically noticeable where the patient is now concerned by the cosmesis, which they previously found tolerable. If the deviation is large enough to be cosmetically distressing then few of these cases will be likely to be treatable in optometric practice and most will require referral for a surgeon's opinion.

Other cases of long-standing strabismus might request treatment for vocational reasons: the patient might now wish to pursue a career that requires orthotropia, or better vision in an amblyopic eye. For reasons outlined earlier in this chapter, the treatment of these cases is associated with a risk of diplopia and treatment should only be attempted by practitioners who are experienced and knowledgeable in orthoptic techniques.

One particular type of strabismus requires specific mention in this section: infantile esotropia syndrome. This type of strabismus occurs in the first 6 months of life and this early-onset interruption to the development of binocularity usually has lasting consequences. Two of these consequences can be confusing when they are encountered and these are **latent nystagmus** and **dissociated vertical deviation**. Latent nystagmus is horizontal nystagmus which is either only present or is greatly exaggerated by monocular occlusion (see Chapter 7). Dissociated vertical deviation typically gives the appearance of an alternating hyperphoria. When either eye is covered, the eye behind the cover moves upwards. The eye may even start to move upwards as the cover approaches, before the eye is actually covered. These patients will typically have a history of a large angle esotropia in early life that usually has been surgically corrected.

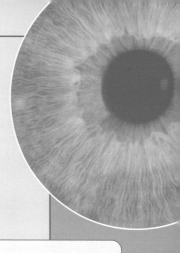

4
Microtropia

What is microtropia?

Microtropia is defined in different ways by various authors. To many, microtropia simply means a small angle strabismus: often defined as less than 10Δ or sometimes as less than 6Δ. Many different factors are typically associated with microtropia, and these are listed in Table 4.1. Some authors define microtropia according to some of these associated factors. An example of this is "microtropia with identity". This is a microtropia when the angle of eccentric fixation is the same as the angle of the strabismus. This means that no strabismic movement (see Table 1.1) is seen on cover testing: indeed, a movement may be seen which looks

Table 4.1 Algorithm for the diagnosis of microtropia. Reproduced with permission from Evans, 2002, *Pickwell's Binocular Vision Anomalies*, 4th edition, Butterworth-Heinemann

All the following characteristics must be present for a diagnosis of microtropia

- Angle less than 10Δ
- Amblyopic eye with morphoscopic acuity at least one line worse than non-amblyoptic eye, unless alternating microtropia (rare)
- Eccentric fixation, unless alternating microtropia (rare)
- HARC detected by Bagolini striated lens test, or by Modified Mallett OXO Test

And at least three of the following characteristics should also be present

- Angle less than 6Δ
- Anisometropia over 1.50D
- Microtropia with identity: angle of anomaly = angle of eccentric fixation, so no movement when dominant eye is covered
- Monofixational syndrome: apparent phoria movement on cover test
- Motor fusion: "pseudo-fusional reserves" can be measured
- Stereopsis of 100″ or more on contoured (monocularly visible) tests such as Titmus circles, or Randot contoured circles
- Four prism diopter test shows positive response (the absence of the normal movement)
- Lang's one-sided scotoma demonstrated with Amsler charts

like heterophoria. Some authors only use the term microtropia to describe these cases of microtropia with identity. Other authors say that microtropia just means a small angle strabismus, and to these authors microtropia with identity is just one particular type (subdivision) of microtropia.

An attempt has been made to bring these different viewpoints together in Table 4.1. The features that are almost universally accepted as present in every case of microtropia are listed in the first part of the table. The second part of the table lists features which are commonly present in microtropia. In Table 4.1 these factors are given a hierarchy to create a diagnostic algorithm for microtropia.

How do I investigate?

Table 4.1 summarizes the investigation of microtropia. Most cases of microtropia will have amblyopia and this should be investigated as detailed in Chapter 5. The detection of HARC is summarized in Chapter 3.

The cases that are hardest to investigate are microtropia with identity, when no sign of the strabismus will be seen on cover testing. These cases may present as unexplained poor acuity in one eye. There may be anisometropia, in which case the differential diagnosis is between pure anisometropic amblyopia and, if a microtropia is present, mixed strabismic and anisometropic amblyopia. It can be important to make this differential diagnosis in patients who are keen to pursue treatment of their amblyopia. This is because patching can be tried in adults with pure anisometropic amblyopia but should not be attempted in adults with strabismic amblyopia (see Chapter 5). In these cases, many of the tests in Table 4.1 will help with the differential diagnosis, but the most useful tests are to look for eccentric fixation with the ophthalmoscope (see Table 5.4) and to test for central suppression. Unfortunately, the standard test for suppression in microtropia, the 4Δ base out test, does not always give conclusive results. This is probably because too little attention is paid to the fixation target. The assumption behind the test is that a 4Δ base out prism in front of a microtropic eye will move a fixation target within the central suppression area, so an eye movement will not occur. For this test to work, an isolated target should be used. Practitioners often use a letter on a Snellen chart, but, of course, the whole chart will be displaced by the 4Δ lens, not just the fixation letter. A suggested method of use for the 4Δ base out test is summarized in Table 4.2.

Table 4.2   Method of use of the 4Δ base out test

1. The theory behind the test is that in a microtropic eye there is likely to be a central suppression area. This means that if a target is displaced by a 4Δ prism then the strabismic eye is unlikely to make an appropriate eye movement because the target will be displaced within the central suppression area
2. Select an appropriate target, which should be an isolated target on a large uniform field. A dot (perceivable by the amblyopic eye) on a white, otherwise featureless, wall in front of the patient is ideal. A dot in the center of a blank sheet of A3 or A4 paper is also acceptable
3. Introduce the 4Δ base out lens in front of one eye whilst the eyes fixate the target
4. If the patient has no strabismus then one of two normal responses, or a combination of both, will occur: a. both eyes will make a saccadic version movement, followed by a vergence movement of the eye without the prism, or b. the eye with the prism will make a vergence movement, the other eye maintaining fixation
5. If the patient has a microtropia and the prism is placed in front of the strabismic eye then the image will be displaced within the central suppression area and no movement of either eye will take place
6. If the patient has a microtropia and the prism is placed in front of the non-strabismic eye then both eyes will make a saccadic version movement, but there will be no corrective vergence movement
7. If an abnormal response is obtained, then the better (normal) eye should be occluded and the test repeated with the prism just introduced in front of the monocularly fixing eye. If this eye still fails to make a saccadic movement to the prism then this suggests that pathology may be present, causing a central scotoma

Results with the 4Δ base out test can be inconclusive, and it is best not to base the diagnosis of microtropia on this test alone. The test is meant to detect central suppression and the foveal suppression test described in Table 2.4 may be a better test. In any event, the best method of diagnosing a complex condition like microtropia is to combine the results of several tests, as suggested in Table 4.1.

When do I need to do something?

With the exception of amblyopia (see Chapter 5), the answer to this question is hardly ever! Microtropia has been described as a "fully adapted strabismus" and if a patient is fully adapted to a condition then that condition is unlikely to require treatment. One of the features that favors the development of HARC (Table 3.1) is a small angle and nearly all cases (some authors would say all cases) of microtropia have deep HARC and are asymptomatic. This HARC will often allow "pseudo-binocularity": there may be no sign of a strabismus on cover testing and pseudo-convergence, pseudo-fusional reserves and even pseudo-stereopsis may be present.

What do I do?

As mentioned above, most cases of microtropia do not require treatment. Unless the patient has symptoms, it is best to do as little as possible to interfere with the patient's current status. If there is a prism or decentration in the glasses, then it is best to replicate this in any new glasses. If any anisometropia is only partly corrected, then do not make large changes to the degree to which this is corrected.

If the patient is desperate to improve their binocular status, then a few practitioners with particular experience in this field might consider treatment (see pp. 55–56). Treatment of these cases is not without risk (principally, of diplopia) and should only be undertaken by experienced practitioners who can monitor the patient appropriately.

Very rarely, practitioners might encounter a patient with microtropia who has symptoms. It is possible that this could result from the microtropia decompensating into a larger angle strabismus. The "pseudo-binocularity" of microtropia can decompensate in much the same way as true binocularity can decompensate. If the factors that are causing the decompensation can be identified and treated then the condition will be helped. For more specific treatment, the caveats in the preceding paragraph will apply. If the angle of deviation is changing then the reason for this must be known, or the patient must be referred so that this reason can be determined.

5
Amblyopia

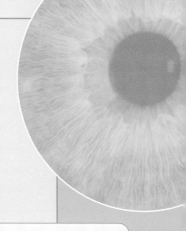

What is amblyopia?

Amblyopia has been defined as a visual loss resulting from an impediment or disturbance to the normal development of vision. It usually exists when an early interruption to the development of vision causes a visual deficit which, in later life, cannot be corrected refractively.

There is a **sensitive period** during which the visual system is still capable of developing amblyopia. For humans, this is said to extend until the age of about 7–8 years. During this period, any interruption to binocularity or to a clear image in one or both eyes is likely to cause amblyopia. There is no abrupt ending to the sensitive period: in reality, disruption to the visual system becomes progressively less likely to cause amblyopia as the child ages and the likelihood of this happening is close to zero by about the age of 8 years.

Amblyopia can be broadly classified into organic and functional. Organic amblyopia results from some pathological abnormality, such as retinal eye disease or toxic factors. Organic amblyopia is rare and practitioners are much more likely to encounter functional amblyopia. The classification of functional amblyopia is summarized in Figure 5.1. Stimulus deprivation amblyopia (e.g., from congenital cataract) and strabismic amblyopia used to collectively be called amblyopia ex anopsia, but this term is seldom used nowadays. The two most common forms of

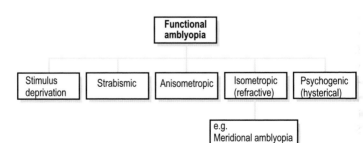

Figure 5.1 Classification of functional amblyopia

amblyopia are strabismic and anisometropic, and these two types have rather different characteristics. Strabismic and anisometropic amblyopia often co-exist, when the characteristics of the amblyopia are best considered as strabismic amblyopia.

Isometropic amblyopia occurs when both eyes have an amblyogenic refractive error (e.g., high astigmatism or high hypermetropia). Hysterical amblyopia is a form of visual conversion reaction and is discussed below.

Two quantitative approaches are commonly used to diagnose amblyopia: a difference between the best corrected acuity of the two eyes of two lines or more and/or acuity in the amblyopic eye of less than 6/9 (assuming that the child is old enough for the visual acuity norms to be 6/6). Additionally, the person should show no sign of another condition (e.g., pathology) that might account for the reduced vision.

The prevalence of amblyopia is about 3%. The vast majority of cases of amblyopia are either strabismic or anisometropic or both. There is some debate over whether strabismic or anisometropic amblyopia is more common, with some studies suggesting that they are equally prevalent.

How do I investigate?

Visual acuity assessment in pre-school children

Amblyopia is initially detected as reduced visual acuity and, for strabismic amblyopia, the visual acuity is much worse for crowded than for isolated targets. Since one of the main goals of measuring visual acuity in young children is to detect strabismic amblyopia, it follows that crowded targets should wherever possible be used when measuring the vision of young children. By the age of about 4–5 years nearly all children can match letters on a Snellen chart with similar letters on a matching card and this type of acuity test is the goal. As soon as letters can be recognized then a proper Snellen test can be conducted.

For children aged 2–4 years, various "crowded" acuity charts are available, which usually come with matching cards. A range of

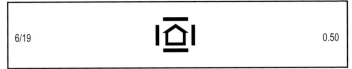

6/19   0.50

Figure 5.2   Lea Symbols Test, as presented in crowded format with the computerized Test Chart 2000 (reproduced with permission from Thomson Software Solutions)

such tests are available with the computerized Test Chart 2000 (Figure 5.2), which has the advantage of allowing optotypes to be randomized. This is especially important for monitoring the effects of amblyopia treatment, since it prevents children from memorizing the test charts. One of the limitations of conventional Snellen charts is a very limited number of optotypes for lower acuities (e.g., only two optotypes on most 6/24 lines), and this greatly increases the risk of children memorizing a certain line. It may be necessary to periodically check the vision in a different consulting room to guard against this.

The Lea Symbols Test (Figure 5.2) can be made into a matching or naming "game" and can be used to obtain binocular acuities with most children from about the age of 2 years. Of course, monocular testing is important for detecting amblyopia, but this can be problematic for some children around the age of 2–3 years who object to occlusion. In some cases, occlusion for visual acuity testing is just not possible and the best that can be done is to see if the child is equally unhappy to have either eye occluded, which suggests approximately equal acuity. The child should be tested frequently (e.g., every 3–4 months) until monocular visual acuities can be recorded, which is nearly always possible in the third year of life. If a child refuses to have one eye covered, but quite happily tolerates occlusion of the other eye, then this is a highly suspicious sign and might suggest poor vision in the eye that is uncovered when they object most. If good results are not obtained with such a child, then a cycloplegic or very early retest is indicated. If there is any doubt about such cases then they should be referred.

Below the age of about 2 years, preferential looking tests may be required, such as the Cardiff acuity test. This works well for children aged 1–2 years, but is not good at detecting strabismic amblyopia. This is why crowded tests with pictures or letters should be used as soon as possible (e.g., Figure 5.2).

Typical tests for different ages with typical results are given in Table 5.1. As one might expect, different tests produce results that are not perfectly equivalent, so the figures in Table 5.1 are an approximation. To give maximum clinical validity, it is important to test patients with standard letter charts as soon as they can cope with these. In vision screening programs it is important to have a strict criterion and every child who achieves below this level would be referred. In a primary care eye examination the situation is rather different and so the values in Table 5.1 are only for guidance, since other factors will need to be taken into consideration. For example, a significant refractive error, symptoms or reduced vision in solely one eye will raise the index of suspicion.

Table 5.1 Approximate minimum levels of visual acuity with different tests for various ages. Note: measurements are notoriously variable in children, so different authors often quote quite markedly different norms

Age	Test	Approximate norms
0–1 year	Keeler preferential looking cards	• 3 months: 6/90 • 6 months: 6/30 • 12 months: 6/24
1–3 years	Cardiff acuity cards	• 12 months: 6/38 • 24 months: 6/15 • 36 months: 6/12
3–5 years	Lea Symbols Crowded Test Kay Crowded Picture Test LogMAR Crowded Test (Glasgow Acuity Cards) Cambridge Crowded Cards Snellen matching	• 36 months: 6/12 • 48 months: 6/9 • 60 months: 6/7.5
Over 5 years	Snellen	• 6/7.5

Differentially diagnosing amblyopia and reduced vision from pathology

Amblyopia is detected as reduced vision in one eye. Potentially, reduced vision can result from pathology so an important part of the investigation of amblyopia is to rule out pathology. There are two approaches to this, both of which must be followed in every case: the practitioner must obtain a **negative sign** and a **positive sign**. The negative sign is the exclusion of pathology (Table 5.2). The second step is to look for amblyogenic factors and to obtain a positive sign of at least one of these (Table 5.3).

Excluding pathology in the differential diagnosis of amblyopia (Table 5.2) is not a "one off" activity. It is rare in the healthcare sciences that a diagnosis is absolutely certain: at every appointment the practitioner should keep an open mind, review their diagnosis, and be prepared to change their mind if the findings so indicate.

Differentially diagnosing strabismic and anisometropic amblyopia

There are differences between the treatment of strabismic amblyopia and anisometropic amblyopia (see below). So, the differential diagnosis of these two types of amblyopia is important. This is problematic in microtropia, which can be difficult to detect and may show no movement on cover testing (see Chapter 4). In these cases the detection of eccentric fixation, which is usually present in strabismic amblyopia, can be a helpful diagnostic sign. There are various methods of detecting eccentric fixation, but these days overwhelmingly the most popular technique is to use the direct ophthalmoscope. The method for this is summarized in Table 5.4 and a suggested method of recording is given in Figure 5.3.

When do I need to do something?

Amblyopia is commonly inherited, so when an eye examination is carried out and amblyopia is detected then one important action

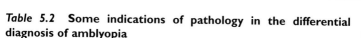

Table 5.2 Some indications of pathology in the differential diagnosis of amblyopia

Step	What to do
Detect any ocular pathology	• Check pupil reactions, particularly looking for an APD • Carry out careful ophthalmoscopy. In younger children, dilated fundoscopy might be necessary to obtain a good view, commonly after cycloplegic refraction. Keep checking ophthalmoscopy at regular intervals • As soon as the child is old enough, check visual fields
Look for neurological problems	• Carefully check pupil reactions • Assess and record optic disc appearance in both eyes, if possible with photographs • Look for incomitancy and/or strabismus (may be a sign of neurological problems) • As soon as the child is old enough, check visual fields • Monitor reports of general health (e.g., neurological signs, including headache)
Is the amblyopia responding to treatment?	• If amblyopia that is being treated at an appropriate age does not respond to treatment, then review the diagnosis • Failure to respond to treatment might indicate a pathological cause, so refer for a second opinion • If the visual acuity in a presumed amblyopic eye worsens, then it is probably something other than amblyopia and requires early referral for further investigation

is necessary, regardless of the age of the patient. This is to advise the patient that any close family members who are children should have a full eye examination, as young as possible. If the

Table 5.3 **Detecting amblyogenic factors in the differential diagnosis of amblyopia. The presence of an amblyogenic factor does not mean that pathology cannot be present and the factors in Table 5.2 still need to be considered**

Step	Rationale	What to do
Detect strabismus	If there is a strabismic eye with reduced vision, then the patient probably has strabismic amblyopia	1. Carry out a careful cover test (Table 1.1) • Test for microtropia (Table 4.1) • Look for incomitancy (Chapter 6) • Look for eccentric fixation (see below)
Look for anisometropia	If the patient has anisometropia and the eye with the higher refractive error has reduced VA, then the patient probably has anisometropic amblyopia	• Carry out a careful refraction • Cycloplegic refraction (or Mohindra retinoscopy) may be necessary
Look for other refractive errors	Isometropic amblyopia is rarer, but can occur in high bilateral uncorrected refractive errors	• Carry out a careful refraction • Cycloplegic refraction (or Mohindra retinoscopy) may be necessary

patient is a child, then the aim is to detect siblings. If the patient is an adult, then the aim is to detect children or grandchildren. The standards of children's vision screening programs are variable, so this advice should be given regardless of any screening that the child may undergo.

There are fundamental differences between the characteristics of anisometropic and strabismic amblyopia. For people with anisometropia and strabismus, the amblyopia bears the characteristics of strabismic amblyopia and these people should be classified in this way. Isometropic amblyopia can probably be thought of as "bilateral anisometropic amblyopia".

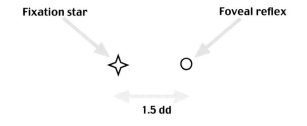

Fixation star **Foveal reflex**

1.5 dd

Fixation slightly unstable compared with dominant eye

Figure 5.3 Suggested method of recording eccentric fixation. It is important to label the foveal reflex and the fixation target. The degree of eccentric fixation can be recorded, using a disc diameter (dd) or drawing the ophthalmoscope graticule (if present) as the unit of measurement. If the ophthalmoscope graticule is used then record the make and model of ophthalmoscope. There may be a slight vertical element to the eccentric fixation

Strabismic amblyopia

The sensitive period for the development of amblyopia was discussed above. For strabismic amblyopia, there is also a sensitive period for the treatment of amblyopia. If strabismic amblyopia is treated before the age of about 7–12 years then treatment is much more likely to be effective than after this age. Over the age of 7–12 years, there is another reason why treatment is contraindicated in addition to the decreased likelihood of success. This is because of the binocular sensory adaptations to strabismus (HARC or global suppression; Chapter 3), which are very likely to be present in cases of strabismus which develop before 7–12 years of age. Although these binocular sensory adaptations are distinctly different from amblyopia, the binocular sensory adaptations might nonetheless be "broken down" by prolonged periods of treatment. This could cause diplopia. For these two reasons (low likelihood of success and risk of diplopia), it is usually recommended that strabismic amblyopia should not be treated over the age of 7–12 years, and should only be treated in this age range with caution (p. 77). Therefore, the period up to

Table 5.4 Method of using the direct ophthalmoscope to test for eccentric fixation

1. If the consulting room is not completely dark, then the eye that is not being tested should be occluded
2. First, test the eye with **better** visual acuity. This serves to train the patient and to check their response
3. Select the ophthalmoscope fixation target (usually a star, sometimes with a measuring graticule)
4. With the room lights turned out or dimmed, project this target onto a surface (e.g., the consulting room ceiling) and point out the fixation target. Explain to the patient that they will see this projected into their eye and, when so instructed, they must fixate the star very precisely, without looking away
5. Initially, instruct the patient to look straight ahead, and not at the fixation star. Look in their eye, find the optic disc, and focus the ophthalmoscope in the usual way
6. Once the ophthalmoscope is focused, ask the patient to look at the star as precisely and steadily as possible
7. Note how central and steady is their fixation. Since this is the non-amblyopic eye, the fixation should be central and steady. Record the results
8. Now, repeat steps 5–7 but in the eye with **worse** acuity. Record the result

the age of 7–12 years can be thought of as the "window of opportunity" for treating strabismic amblyopia.

The impression is sometimes given of a fairly abrupt end to the sensitive period for treatment at about the seventh birthday. Of course, this oversimplification is unlikely to be accurate. Neural plasticity probably gradually diminishes throughout life and the 7–12-year-old guide above is bound to be approximate. If this gradual decline in neural plasticity is true, then it follows that it is likely to be better to treat strabismic amblyopia at as young an age as possible. All this means that primary eyecare practitioners must be capable of detecting strabismic amblyopia and when they do detect it under the age of 7–12 years then they must do something about it. Specifically, they must either treat it themselves or refer it to someone else for treatment.

Anisometropic amblyopia

The treatment of anisometropic amblyopia is an interesting example of the situation where the scientific literature tells a rather different story to the clinical "received wisdom". It is often stated, sometimes even in textbooks, that anisometropic amblyopia must, like strabismic amblyopia, be treated before age 7–12 years. However, the scientific evidence suggests that there is no such sensitive period for anisometropic amblyopia. For cases of pure anisometropic amblyopia (i.e., when there is no strabismus) treatment can be attempted at any age. Most studies have failed to find a significant effect of age on treatment: treatment is almost as effective in adults as it is in younger children. It seems implausible that there is no effect of age at all, but the effect is certainly weak.

What do I do?

As noted above, strabismic amblyopia and anisometropic amblyopia need to be considered differently. If a patient has anisometropia and strabismus (common in microtropia) then the patient should be treated as a strabismic amblyope.

The treatment of amblyopia, particularly patching, is not without disadvantages. Whilst the patch is worn the child will be forced to live with reduced vision, and the psycho-social consequences of patching (e.g., disruption to the child's quality of life) are a cause for concern. As always, the decision to treat should only be made after due discussion with the parent and (if old enough) the child. In a given case, the disadvantages of patching need to be weighed against the chances of success, which will depend on several factors (e.g., age, degree of any anisometropia, etc.). But although patching is never popular, the risk of the person losing sight in their good eye in later life (e.g., from injury or AMD) cannot be ignored and is a powerful reason to treat.

Strabismic amblyopia

In strabismic amblyopia the strabismus may need treatment, as outlined in Chapter 3. The present section just deals with amblyopia, and the management of this will differ for different age groups, as detailed below. The most important advice when seeing a patient with strabismic amblyopia who is within the sensitive period is to do something and to do this decisively. Either the patient should be treated, or referred to someone else to treat. If they are treated, the parents/child should be given clear instructions and monitored frequently.

Under age 3 years

These cases are difficult to manage in a primary care setting, unless the practice has specialist facilities for pre-school children (e.g., Keeler acuity cards) and is experienced in dealing with this age group. Generally, it is best to refer to a primary eyecare colleague or hospital department who have the appropriate equipment and expertise. If patients of this age are to be treated, then a fairly typical procedure is outlined in Table 5.5.

Age 3–7 years

Children aged 3–7 years can usually be treated in most community optometric practices, or in hospital departments. For children in this age range, occlusion amblyopia is less of a worry and steps 2–10 in Table 5.5 are usually followed. With older children in this age range, alternative methods of occlusion will be more acceptable to the patient, such as a "pirate-type" patch, a frosted lens on glasses, a spectacle lens or contact lens of an inappropriate power, or cyclopentolate penalization. The essential feature is that the good eye is occluded or blurred to an acuity that is significantly worse than the amblyopic eye. Some of these alternative forms of occlusion make it easier for the child to "cheat", for example by tilting their head so that they are looking round a frosted spectacle lens. These forms of occlusion are only appropriate if the practitioner is confident that the parent is willing to monitor the child carefully for these signs.

Table 5.5 **Method for treating strabismic amblyopia in children under the age of 3 years**

1.	For these young children there is a significant risk of causing occlusion amblyopia: amblyopia of the occluded eye. To prevent this, the usual advice is to occlude the good eye for one day per year of age, then patch the other eye for one day; and then repeat the cycle. For example, in a 2-year-old the good eye would be patched for 2 days, then the amblyopic eye for one day, and so on
2.	Amblyopia treatment can only be fully effective if there is a clear image. Appropriate refractive correction for the amblyopic eye is essential
3.	Total occlusion is generally recommended, usually with an adhesive patch
4.	Full time occlusion is also usually recommended, but with the patch removed for any tasks when normal vision is needed for safety (e.g., riding a bike in older children)
5.	Explain to the parent how the child might "cheat" (e.g., lifting edge of patch and turning head). Children cannot be blamed for trying to use their better eye, but patching will only work if the parent detects and stops any cheating
6.	The patient should be encouraged to do tasks that involve detailed vision. For example, playing with small toys or watching a favorite television program or video. To begin with, encourage the parents to give the child a "treat" when the patch is put on
7.	Careful monitoring is required, typically 3 weeks after treatment starts and regularly thereafter. In addition to monitoring acuities in the amblyopic and non-strabismic eye, the parent's observations should also be recorded and cover test, motility and periodically ophthalmoscopy and retinoscopy repeated
8.	If the acuity does not improve significantly (e.g., by a line on the LogMAR Crowded Test) then re-evaluate the diagnosis (see Table 5.2)
9.	Occlusion is continued until there has been no further improvement over 5–6 weeks
10.	The patient is then monitored every few months to ensure that the acuity in the strabismic eye does not "drop back". If so, re-instigate treatment

Depending on the starting acuity, with older children it might be decided to postpone treatment until the school holidays, if occlusion would make their acuity so poor that it would cause them to fall behind at school. If this is the case, then part-time occlusion might be tried whilst watching television until the holidays when full-time occlusion could be started. Indeed, recent research suggests that treatment is effective for "dose rates" of 2 hours a day or more, but greater dose rates reduce the number of weeks necessary to achieve the best acuity.

It is important to fully explain the goals of treatment to both the parent and the child. Most children can understand the concept of exercising a weak eye so as to make it stronger. Children in this age range often enjoy video games and these can be a great source of motivation. Encourage the child and parent to keep a score of the good eye performance at the test and to compare this with the "bad eye". Each day they play the game with the bad eye and try to improve the score. Sometimes, a graph of the best score each day for the bad eye will help the child to visualize it improving. Of course, parents must ensure that the child keeps a reasonable distance away from the screen.

Aged 7–12 years

As noted on p. 71, there is a concern about treating this age group since it is possible that treatment might cause a binocular sensory adaptation (HARC or global suppression) to break down. So, the binocular sensory adaptation will need to be carefully monitored during treatment and part-time occlusion is usually felt to be more appropriate than full-time. In view of the slight risk of intractable diplopia, many practitioners do not treat this age group and less-experienced practitioners may feel happier referring these cases to colleagues. But referral should be prompt since unnecessary delay at this age should be avoided.

Anisometropic amblyopia

A typical approach to treating anisometropic amblyopia is outlined in Table 5.6. Anisometropic amblyopia is a refractive problem, so accurate refractive correction is at the core of the

Table 5.6 Method for treating anisometropic (non-strabismic) amblyopia

1.	Prescribe refractive correction, fully correcting the degree of anisometropia (usually revealed by cycloplegic refraction)
2.	Check the patient after about 4–6 weeks. If there has been a significant (typically, one line or more) improvement, then continue with refractive correction alone until the amblyopic eye either (a) stops improving or (b) the acuity of the amblyopic eye equals that of the better eye
3.	If (a) occurs before (b) then proceed to occlusion
4.	Occlusion can only be fully effective if there is a clear image. So, occlusion must be used with the appropriate refractive correction
5.	Total occlusion is generally recommended, usually with an adhesive patch. If the acuity is not too bad (e.g., 6/12 or better) and the patient old enough not to "cheat" then more cosmetically acceptable forms of patch (e.g., frosted lens in spectacles) can be used
6.	In anisometropic amblyopia, the occlusion should **not** be full time since periods of normal binocular vision may be required to maintain binocularity. There should be at least 2 h a day without the occluder. Typically, the occlusion is started for about 4–6 hours a day and then increased if the improvement in acuity is slow
7.	If patients have a large heterophoria or one that has signs of being close to decompensation (see Chapter 2) then they should only be occluded for brief periods, starting with 1 hour and gradually increasing if the heterophoria remains compensated (see point 10 below)
8.	Explain to the parent how the child might "cheat" (e.g., lifting edge of patch and turning head). Children cannot be blamed for trying to use their better eye, but patching will only work if the parent detects and stops any cheating
9.	The patient should be encouraged to do tasks that involve detailed vision. For example, playing with small toys or watching a favorite television program or video. To begin with, encourage the parents to give the child a "treat" when the patch is put on

10. Patients should be warned to look out for diplopia and parents to look out for a turning eye when they remove the patch. If this occurs, then they should stop patching and return for their binocularity to be checked to ensure that any heterophoria is not decompensating (see Chapter 2)

11. Careful monitoring is required, typically 4–6 weeks after treatment starts and regularly thereafter. In addition to monitoring acuities in both eyes, the parent's observations should also be recorded and cover test, motility, stereopsis, and periodically ophthalmoscopy and retinoscopy repeated

12. If the acuity does not improve significantly (e.g., by a line on the LogMAR Crowded Test) then re-evaluate the diagnosis (see Table 5.2)

13. Occlusion is continued until there has been no further improvement over 5–6 weeks

14. The patient is then monitored every few months to ensure that the acuity in the strabismic eye does not "drop back". In anisometropic amblyopia this is unlikely

treatment. Optically, the best form of refractive correction is contact lenses. For older children and adults this can be suggested, if other factors (e.g., personal hygiene) are suitable. Unlike the standard use of contact lenses by myopes, anisometropic amblyopes do not perceive an immediate advantage on insertion of their contact lenses. This makes it more likely that they will drop out of wearing daily wear contact lenses. Silicone hydrogel continuous wear contact lenses can be a good solution for suitable cases because they don't have to remember to insert the lenses every day.

If occlusion is necessary, then the procedure is as outlined in steps 4–14 in Table 5.6. For older children, the same motivating approaches employing video games can be used as outlined in the preceding section.

It is not uncommon to encounter adults with previously uncorrected anisometropia, or with anisometropia that has only been partly corrected. If these patients are asymptomatic and happy to carry on as they are then this may be the best course of action. But it is possible that any amblyopia might reduce with appropriate refractive correction, possibly with additional patching. If the anisometropia is high (over 3–4D), then appropriate refractive correction is likely to mean contact lenses or refractive surgery. Indeed, through reducing aniseikonia, contact lenses or refractive surgery are likely to be the best modes of correction for all cases of anisometropia, and therefore will increase the chances of the vision improving without the patient requiring occlusion. In pure (non-strabismic) cases of anisometropic amblyopia, occlusion can be attempted in adults, but this is usually only carried out for brief periods (e.g., 30 minutes) of detailed use of the amblyopic eye. Patients should be monitored closely and warned as noted in point 10 of Table 5.6.

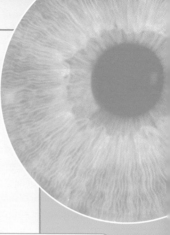

6

Incomitant deviations

What is an incomitant deviation?

An incomitant deviation is a deviation whose angle varies in different positions of gaze and depending on which eye is fixing. Incomitancy can be congenital or can be acquired. An incomitancy can be stable for years and then decompensate. The decompensation can occur for a reason, such as ill health or the patient being forced to look in a direction that causes them problems for prolonged periods. In other cases, the decompensation can occur without any apparent reason.

Most incomitant deviations can be broadly classified as neurogenic or mechanical. Neurogenic incomitancies are caused by some lesion affecting the nervous system and are sub-classified depending on the site of that lesion as supra-nuclear, inter-nuclear or infra-nuclear. Mechanical incomitancies occur as a result of some muscular or orbital lesion that mechanically restricts the movement of the globe.

The etiology of acquired incomitant deviations can be broadly classified as vascular, neurological or "other" (see Table 6.1). The likely etiologies will vary greatly with age. Some etiologies for an acquired incomitancy in an older person are vascular, myasthenia gravis, tumor, trauma (falls) or thyroid eye disease. In young adults trauma (road traffic accidents), migraine or multiple sclerosis are more likely etiologies. Some of the etiologies in Table 6.1 are life-threatening, so a new or changing incomitancy requires urgent referral.

Table 6.1 **Etiology of acquired incomitant deviations**

Vascular	Neurological	Other
Diabetes	Tumor	Trauma
Vascular hypertension	Multiple sclerosis	Thyroid eye disease
Stroke	Migraine	Toxic
Aneurysm	Myasthenia gravis	Iatrogenic
Giant cell arteritis		Idiopathic

The medial and lateral recti are easy to understand and the superior and inferior recti and obliques can be best understood by studying Figure 6.1. If the muscles are imagined to contract whilst looking at this figure, then their actions can be seen to be as indicated in Table 6.2. The mnemonic RADSIN is a useful reminder that the superior and inferior **r**ecti **ad**duct and the superior recti and obliques **in**tort.

A key point to note is that the system is dynamic: the actions of the muscles will change as the globe moves into different positions. This is best understood by viewing Figure 6.1a and imagining the actions of the superior rectus if the globe is turned out by about 23°. Now, the front to back axis of the globe will be exactly the same as the line of pull of the superior rectus. So, when this muscle contracts the globe will be elevated and none of the secondary actions in Table 6.2 will apply. In other words, the information in Table 6.2 only applies to the primary position,

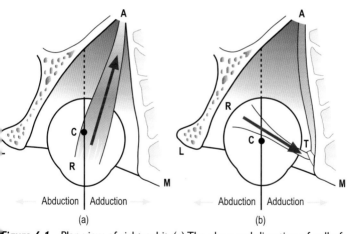

Abduction | Adduction   Abduction | Adduction

(a)   (b)

Figure 6.1 Plan view of right orbit. (a) The plane and direction of pull of the superior and inferior recti muscles, RA, which passes medial (M) to the plane of the center of rotation of the eye (C). (b) The plane containing the superior and inferior oblique muscles; their direction of pull is almost the same. It passes behind and medial to the center of rotation (reproduced with permission from Evans, B.J.W. (2002) *Pickwell's Binocular Vision Anomalies*, 4th edition, Butterworth-Heinemann)

Table 6.2 **Actions of the extra-ocular muscles in the primary position**

Muscle	Primary action	Secondary action	Tertiary action
Medial rectus	Adduction	None	None
Lateral rectus	Abduction	None	None
Superior rectus	Elevation	Intorsion	Adduction
Inferior rectus	Depression	Extorsion	Adduction
Superior oblique	Intorsion	Depression	Abduction
Inferior oblique	Extorsion	Elevation	Abduction

but would be relevant, for example, in interpreting cover test results obtained with the eyes in the primary position.

In ocular motility testing, a goal is to obtain an estimate of the functioning of each extra-ocular muscle. So, the globe needs to be made to look in the position of gaze in which each extra-ocular muscle has its maximum action. For the superior rectus, this will be when the eye looks out and up. The other "principal actions" of the extra-ocular muscles in these cardinal positions of gaze are illustrated in Figure 6.2.

Many patients have an A- or V-syndrome and, in fact, there are a variety of other similar but less common "alphabet syndromes", such as X-, Y- and inverted Y-syndromes. In an A-syndrome the patient is relatively more exo (or less eso) in downgaze than in upgaze. In a V-syndrome they are relatively more exo (or less eso) in upgaze than in downgaze. In some ways these resemble an incomitant deviation, since the deviation varies in different positions of gaze. However, they would not be expected to vary depending on which eye is fixing.

How do I investigate?

The ocular motility test is the most important part of the eye examination for detecting incomitant deviations. It is essential to

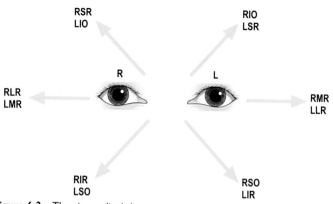

Figure 6.2 The six cardinal diagnostic positions of gaze, indicating the muscles which should have maximum power to maintain the eyes in these directions. The paired synergists (muscles, one from each eye, which act together) are shown (reproduced with permission from Evans, B.J.W. (2002) *Pickwell's Binocular Vision Anomalies*, 4th edition, Butterworth-Heinemann)

carry out this test on every new patient, every time children are seen, if adults present with new symptoms, and periodically over the years as adults are monitored. There are really three different tests that can be carried out during the ocular motility test, and with incomitant patients the situation can be made simpler by performing the test three times to gather these three sets of information. The first of these three tests, **the basic objective ocular motility test**, is described in Table 6.3.

Table 6.3 Procedure for carrying out the basic objective ocular motility test

1. The best target is a point light source, which should be bright enough to allow the corneal reflexes to be clearly seen, but not so bright as to cause blepharospasm. For infants, any target that will catch their attention is recommended

2. The light should be held at about 50 cm from the patient. It should be moved quite slowly, so that it takes about 5 seconds to move from extreme gaze on one side to extreme gaze on the other

(continued)

Table 6.3 Continued

3.	The light should be moved in an arc, as if using an imaginary perimeter bowl
4.	It is easier to observe the eye movements in extreme gaze if no spectacles are worn, but if there is an accommodative strabismus then spectacles should be worn, or the test repeated with and without spectacles
5.	Various authors have preferences for different patterns of movement of the target. The star pattern is often used, but other patterns have been recommended and each has its own merits
6.	The straight up and down (in the midline) positions are often also tested to look for an A or V syndrome
7.	In young children, the head may need to be gently held. With infants, it is best not to hold the head but to move the target very far around the patient so that the eyes are forced to move when the head cannot turn any more
8.	The motility test is performed whilst watching the reflection of the light in the corneae to detect any marked under-actions or over-actions
9.	Any over- or under-actions can be graded from Grade 1 (just detectable) to Grade 5 (extremely noticeable)
10.	Throughout the test, the corneal reflexes of the light are observed. If one disappears, then either the light is misaligned or the patient's view of the light has been obscured (e.g., by the nose). This means that the light has been moved too far: the test should be carried out within the binocular field
11.	In down gaze, patients often need to be asked to keep their eyes as wide open as possible. The lids should only be physically held open if this is the only way that the reflexes can be seen
12.	If any abnormality is observed on this binocular motility test, then each eye is occluded and a monocular motility test carried out in turn

If a marked deviation is present, then this may be revealed by the basic ocular motility test (Table 6.3). However, this method relies on an observation of corneal reflexes and, as noted on

p. 10, this is an inaccurate method of assessing ocular alignment. The cover test is more accurate and can be carried out during ocular motility testing, as outlined in Table 6.4. Cover testing in peripheral gaze is an extremely useful test and, like the basic ocular motility test, provides objective data. It requires practice, but is well worth the time that it takes to become skilled at this test.

Table 6.4 **Procedure for cover testing in peripheral gaze during the ocular motility test**

1. A point light source is usually used, although in deviations with a significant accommodative element an accommodative target is better
2. An advantage of using a light is that binocular fixation can be monitored (see point 10 in Table 6.3). It is pointless to carry out a cover test if one eye's view of the target is already obscured by the nose
3. A quick cover/uncover and alternating cover test (see Tables 1.1 and 1.2) is carried out in each cardinal position of gaze. Usually, about 4–6 covers are required. Either the size of deviation can be estimated (see Table 1.3) or measured with prisms
4. Care must be taken to ensure that the occluder does fully occlude: it will need to be angled as the target is moved into peripheral gaze
5. The result is recorded as illustrated in Figure 6.3

An even more sensitive way of detecting incomitancy is to use the patient's own visual system to provide feedback on ocular alignment through determining the subjective angle in different positions of gaze. This is made easier by the use of red and green goggles, and this approach is described in Table 6.5. Although with some patients this can be extremely informative, with others it can be a source of considerable confusion. Patients may become dissociated as the test progresses, may be confused about diplopia, or may suppress in certain positions of gaze. Data from the three approaches summarized in Tables 6.3–6.5 should be weighted in the order in which the tables appear.

Table 6.5 Procedure for assessing the subjective angle of deviation in different positions of gaze

1. For patients who do not experience diplopia, red and green goggles are required. Ideally, a bar light and goggles should be used since this allows torsional deviations to be assessed, but this equipment is no longer generally available

2. Patients who experience diplopia can do the test without red or green goggles. However, goggles still help in these cases to readily identify which image belongs to which eye

3. The patient is asked to indicate the relative positions of the two images in different positions of gaze. In its simplest form, this test consists of just drawing the relative positions of these images in the different boxes for different positions of gaze. This usually allows the position of gaze in which there is maximum diplopia to be clearly identified, which greatly assists in the diagnosis of an under-acting muscle

4. Ideally, prisms can be used to bring the two images together and the deviation measured

The motility test results can be recorded as suggested in Figure 6.3. This is particularly useful for the methods described in Tables 6.4 and 6.5. The most important part of this diagram is the key to right gaze and left gaze. Usually, the chart is recorded as shown in Figure 6.3, as if projected from the patient in the same way as the visual field (and Hess plots) are represented. But this is opposite to Figure 6.2, which is a more intuitive way of recording the results for the practitioner who faces the patient whilst carrying out motility testing. As long as the chart is clearly labeled, then the practitioner can record the result whichever way they want.

It is useful to continue this analogy between ocular motility testing and visual field testing. The basic motility test (Table 6.3) is rather akin to confrontation testing and recording diplopia in different positions of gaze (Table 6.5) is more similar to using a Bjerrum screen. A much better method, more analogous with automated perimetry, is to carry out a Hess plot. This is now possible using the computerized Hess Chart developed by

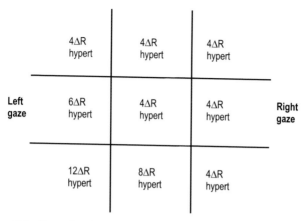

	Left gaze			Right gaze
	4ΔR hypert	4ΔR hypert	4ΔR hypert	
	6ΔR hypert	4ΔR hypert	4ΔR hypert	
	12ΔR hypert	8ΔR hypert	4ΔR hypert	

Figure 6.3 Example of method of recording objective (cover test in peripheral gaze) or subjective deviation in the cardinal positions of gaze. The results are suggestive of a right superior oblique palsy. Note: it is important to label right gaze and left gaze (see text). Hypert., hypertropia

Prof David Thomson at City University. A typical plot, showing a long-standing right superior oblique underaction, is shown in Figure 6.4. Just as with a suspicious visual field plot, the practitioner can retest the patient with the computerized Hess screen after a few weeks to make sure that the situation is not worsening.

It will be noted that with the Hess screen two plots are taken: one with the patient fixing with the right eye and the other when they are fixing with the left eye. This is related to the second half of the definition of incomitancy on p. 82: the deviation will change depending on which eye is fixating. The deviation is larger when the patient is fixating with the paretic eye (the secondary deviation) than when they are fixating with the non-paretic eye (the primary deviation).

If a Hess screen test is not available, or if an additional method of confirming the diagnosis is required, then there are a variety of other diagnostic algorithms. These are designed to help differentially diagnose the cyclo-vertical incomitancies, since these present the greatest challenge. The best known of these is Parks three step and this and an alternative, Scobee's method, are

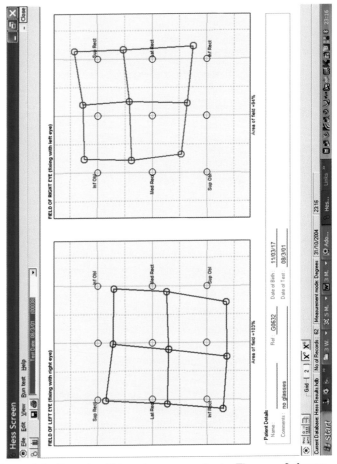

Figure 6.4 Example of Hess plot generated using Thomson Software Solutions Hess Screen. The plot is indicative of a right superior oblique palsy

described in *Pickwell's Binocular Vision Anomalies*, 4th edition. Due to limitations of space, only one of the diagnostic algorithms will be described here and that is Lindblom's method (Table 6.6), which is extremely easy to use and interpret.

Table 6.6 Procedure for Lindblom's method of differentially diagnosing cyclo-vertical incomitancies. The test instructions are given on the left and the paretic muscles indicated by a given answer are on the right

- If the patient has vertical diplopia then they can view, from a distance of 1 m, a 70 cm horizontal wooden rod (if a wooden rod is not available, then a 50 cm or 1 m ruler will suffice)
- If the patient does not have vertical diplopia, then 2 Maddox rods can be used, placed in a trial frame with axes at 90°, so that when the patient views a spotlight at a distance of 1–3 m they see two horizontal red lines

Question 1: Move the wooden rod (or spotlight) up and down and ask: Where is the vertical diplopia (or separation of the red lines) greatest, in up gaze or down gaze?	• Up gaze: RSR, RIO, LSR, LIO • Down gaze: RIR, RSO, LIR, LSO
Question 2: In the position of maximum diplopia, are the two images parallel or torsional?	• Parallel: RSR, RIR, LSR, LIR • Torsional: RSO, RIO, LSO, LIO
Question 3: If parallel, does the separation increase on right or left gaze?	• Right gaze: RSR, RIR • Left gaze: LSR, LIR
Question 4: If tilted, does the illusion of tilt increase in up gaze or down gaze?	• Up gaze: RIO, LIO • Down gaze: RSO, LSO
Question 5: If tilted, then the two rods will resemble an arrow (< or >) or an X. If they resemble an arrow, which way does the arrow point?	The arrow will point to the side with the paretic eye. • Arrow points to right: RSO, RIO • Arrow points to left: LSO, LIO
Question 6: If crossed, does the tilt angle increase in up gaze or down gaze?	• Up gaze: bilateral IO paresis (v. unlikely) • Down gaze: bilateral SO paresis

For Lindblom's method, in cases where the patient does not have diplopia two double Maddox rods need to be used. These should be placed in the cylindrical lens section of a trial frame with the rod axes exactly at 90°, so that the patient perceives two horizontal red lines. This **double Maddox rod test** is informative in itself, quite apart from its role in the Lindblom method. If one of the red lines is tilted then the eye that sees this rod is likely to be the paretic eye and the perceived tilt is in the direction that the affected muscle would rotate the eye. The affected muscle is very likely to be a superior oblique muscle. The trial frame can be adjusted to make the line horizontal and the angle that the rod has to be moved through is equal to the angle of cyclo-deviation. If this is <10° then it suggests that one superior oblique muscle is likely to be paretic; if ≥10° then it is likely to be a bilateral superior oblique paresis. This diagnosis can be confirmed with Lindblom's method, but the axes of the Maddox rod lenses in the trial frame will have to be returned to 90° before the procedure in Table 6.6 is followed.

When do I need to do something?

Long-standing incomitant deviations will not require referral unless they are producing symptoms. This generally only occurs if the incomitancy decompensates, which is rare.

As mentioned above, new or changing incomitancies need to be referred so that any underlying pathology can be detected. Table 6.7 lists the key factors that will aid the differential diagnosis of congenital or long-standing cases from those of recent onset. A new or changing incomitancy is likely to be associated with diplopia, which can be very bothersome to the patient, so temporary occlusion whilst they are awaiting a hospital appointment might be helpful.

What do I do?

The main role of the primary eyecare practitioner is to detect new or changing cases and to refer these. The urgency of referral

Table 6.7 Differential diagnosis of long-standing and recent–onset incomitant deviations

Factor	Congenital or long-standing	Recent onset
Diplopia	Unusual	Usually present in at least one direction of gaze
Onset	Typically, patient does not know when the deviation began	Typically sudden and distressing
Ambylopia	Often present	Absent (almost always)
Comitance	More comitant with time	Typically markedly incomitant
Secondary sequelae	Usually present	Absent, except for overaction of contralateral synergist
Fusion range	May be large in vertical incomitancies	Usually normal
Abnormal head posture (if present)	Slight, but persists on covering paretic eye; patient often unaware of reason for AHP	More marked; the patient is aware of it (to avoid diplopia); disappears on covering paretic eye
Facial asymmetry	May be present	Absent, unless from trauma
Old photographs	May show strabismus or anomalous head posture	Normal
Other symptoms	Unlikely	May be present due to the primary cause

depends on the diagnosis, so this is discussed below. Some long-standing cases have directions of gaze in which they are comfortably binocular, other positions of gaze in which they have a decompensating heterophoria, and other positions in which they are diplopic. It is sometimes possible to help these cases if there is a deviation in the primary position, since correcting this with prisms might increase the field of binocular single and comfortable vision.

The incomitancies that are most likely to be encountered in primary eyecare practices are summarized in Tables 6.8–6.12. The two most common neurogenic incomitancies are lateral rectus palsy and superior oblique palsy. Indeed, it has been said that if a patient presents with diplopia that varies in different positions of gaze, if the diplopia is primarily horizontal then suspect a lateral rectus palsy; if the diplopia is primarily vertical then suspect a

Table 6.8   **Typical features of a superior oblique palsy**

Feature	Detail
Etiology	• Can be congenital • Trauma (quite commonly road traffic accident) • Other etiologies in Table 6.1

Symptoms (if recent onset)	• Diplopia that is predominantly vertical and which is:
	  • possibly described as one image tipped
	  • more marked at near (downgaze) than distance
	  • more marked when looking down and inward (for the affected eye)
	• Also may be symptoms related to the etiology of the palsy

Clinical signs	• Head tilt and/or chin tucked down
	• Hyper-deviation in the affected eye which is larger:
	  • at near than at distance
	  • when looking down and inward (for the affected eye)
	• Underaction of superior oblique on motility testing. In long-standing cases, there can be a variety of secondary sequelae

Management	• If recent onset: urgent referral • If long-standing: varifocals or bifocals are contra-indicated
Additional comments	• A superior oblique palsy can be difficult to detect on motility because: • the main action of the muscle is torsional, which is not assessed on motility testing

- the nose and lids can obstruct the view of the eye when looking down and in
- secondary sequelae may be present
- Secondary sequelae can be particularly confusing with this muscle. Quite commonly, a superior oblique palsy in one eye can lead to a secondary superior rectus palsy in the other eye which, after a number of years, is more marked than the original superior oblique palsy

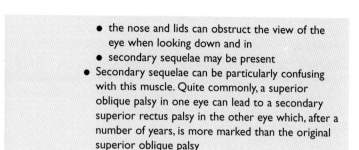

Table 6.9 **Typical features of lateral rectus (sixth nerve) palsy**

Feature	Detail
Etiology	• Can be congenital • Trauma • Vascular (e.g., high blood pressure) • Other etiologies in Table 6.1

Symptoms (if recent onset)	• Head turn
	• Diplopia that is predominantly horizontal and which is:
	  • more marked at distance than near
	  • more marked when looking to the side of the affected muscle
	• Also may be symptoms related to the etiology of the palsy

Clinical signs	• Eso-deviation which is larger:
	  • at distance than near
	  • when looking to the side of the affected muscle
	• Underaction of lateral rectus on motility testing, with overaction of contralateral synergist (medial rectus in the other eye)

Management	• If recent onset: urgent referral • If long-standing: base out prism in distance glasses may help
Additional comments	• It can be difficult to differentially diagnose lateral rectus palsy from one type of Duane's syndrome (see Table 6.11)

Table 6.10 **Typical features of third nerve palsy**

Feature	Detail
Etiology	• Various etiologies in Table 6.1 • The presentation of a third nerve palsy varies greatly: some or all of the muscles served by the third nerve may be affected
Symptoms (if recent onset)	• Diplopia, which in a full third nerve palsy will be constant (although may be ameliorated by ptosis) • Also likely to be symptoms related to the etiology of the palsy
Clinical signs	• In full third nerve palsy, the eye will be down and out with a fixed dilated pupil and ptosis
Management	• If recent-onset total third nerve palsy: emergency referral. Sometimes, a distinction is made between a pupil sparing third nerve palsy (likely to be ischemic, as in diabetes or hypertension) or third nerve palsy where the pupil is dilated (likely to be an aneurysm which could be fatal, so is an emergency). But this distinction is not absolute, so it is safest to refer all cases as an emergency
Additional comments	• This condition is thankfully only rarely seen in primary eyecare practice

superior oblique palsy. It should be noted that there are a variety of incomitant syndromes which are only very rarely encountered in primary eyecare practice. For details of these, more detailed books should be consulted.

A long-standing incomitant deviation can decompensate. If the decompensation is marked, then referral for surgery may be required. If mild, then a prism in the primary position might alleviate the symptoms. Decompensation can be triggered by forcing the person to look into the field of action of the palsied muscle and this is why bifocals or varifocals are contra-indicated in superior oblique palsies (Table 6.8). If a person with an incomitant deviation has binocular single vision in some positions

Table 6.11   Typical features of Duane's syndrome

Feature	Detail
Etiology	• Congenital restrictive anomaly affecting abduction and/or adduction of one or both eye(s)
Symptoms	• Usually, there are no symptoms since the patient compensates with a head turn and/or there is suppression when the person looks in the field of action of the affected muscle
Clinical signs	• Head turn • On motility testing, it is as if one eye is "tethered": • the eye does not move (or barely moves) beyond the horizontal in abduction and/or adduction • there may be up-shoots: an eye aberrantly moves upwards when trying to look to one side • usually, globe retraction is present causing the palpebral aperture to narrow on adduction • There are three types depending on whether abduction, adduction or both are affected. Confusingly, there are two different classifications so it is best to describe the features rather than worrying about the label • Even when the adduction is normal, the near point of convergence is often remote
Management	• If long-standing: no management is usually necessary • If detected in a child and has not been previously investigated: then referral is advisable since there can (rarely) be other associated ocular and/or systemic abnormalities
Additional comments	• This is one of the most common incomitancies seen in primary eyecare practice • In cases where only abduction is affected, it can be difficult to differentially diagnose from a lateral rectus palsy. The presence of palpebral aperture narrowing aids diagnosis, as does a convergence abnormality

Table 6.12   **Typical features of Brown's syndrome**

Feature	Detail
Etiology	• Usually congenital, but can be acquired • Restrictive (mechanical) incomitancy caused by abnormality of the superior oblique tendon sheath which prevents this muscle from feeding out through the trochlea
Symptoms	• Usually there are no symptoms

Clinical signs	• Inability to elevate the eye when adducted
	• In mild cases, this is only apparent when the eye looks up
	• In more marked cases, the affected eye is also hypotropic when attempting adduction without elevation
	• The main challenge is to differentially diagnose the condition from an inferior oblique palsy, which is much rarer. In inferior oblique palsy, there is usually:
	  • an overaction of the superior oblique muscle
	  • a positive Parks 3-steps (or Lindblom's) test
	  • a compensatory head tilt

Management	• If recent onset: urgent referral • If long-standing: usually, no treatment is indicated

of gaze, then this binocularity should be preserved or decompensation could occur. For example, it is probably not advisable to fit these cases with monovision contact lenses.

7
Nystagmus

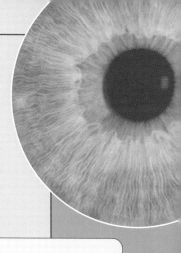

What is nystagmus?

Nystagmus is a regular, repetitive, involuntary movement of the eyes whose direction, amplitude and frequency is variable. It is rare and most commonly has an onset in the first six months of life. The classification of nystagmus is made complicated by various synonyms for the different types, and these are included in parentheses in Figure 7.1.

The two most common types of nystagmus are early-onset nystagmus and latent nystagmus. Early-onset nystagmus occurs in the first six months of life. It may occur secondary to a sensory visual defect (e.g., congenital cataracts, albinism), or

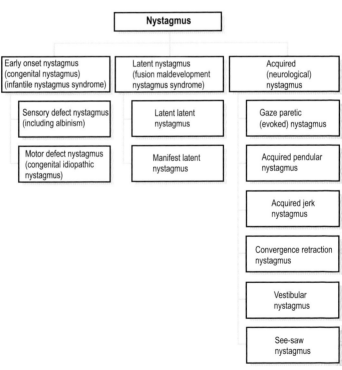

Figure 7.1 Classification of nystagmus

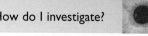

there may be no apparent cause (idiopathic), in which case it is presumed to result from a defect in the motor control of eye movements.

Latent nystagmus becomes much more marked when one eye is covered. In fact, it may not be apparent at all until one eye is covered (latent latent nystagmus); or in other cases it is always present but worsens on occlusion (manifest latent nystagmus). The direction of the nystagmus always reverses when the cover is moved from one eye to the other. Latent nystagmus typically follows an early interruption to the development of binocularity and is most commonly associated with infantile esotropia syndrome. Latent nystagmus therefore occurs early, usually in the first year, of life.

Acquired (neurological) nystagmus can occur at any time, usually after the first few months of life. It is caused by trauma or a lesion (e.g., in multiple sclerosis) affecting the motor pathways.

Two other eye movement anomalies will be mentioned. **Ocular flutter** is a burst of horizontal saccades which can occur in healthy infants, or can result from pathology. About 5% of the population can simulate this effect with **voluntary nystagmus**. **Spasmus nutans** occurs in the first year of life and is characterized by nystagmus, head nodding and abnormal head posture. It is generally benign, but can be associated with pathology.

There are certain problems associated with the evaluation of nystagmus and these are summarized in Table 7.1. The main role for the primary eyecare clinician is to detect the condition, diagnose which of the three main types it is (Figure 7.1), and refer promptly if it is acquired.

How do I investigate?

There are two main aspects to the investigation of nystagmus. First, determine the type of nystagmus and second make a note of the characteristics so that any future change can be detected. The key features of the main types of nystagmus are summarized

Table 7.1 **Problems in the evaluation of nystagmus**

1. Nystagmus is not a condition, but a sign. Many different ocular anomalies can cause nystagmus, or nystagmus can be idiopathic, with no apparent cause

2. Attempts to classify the type of nystagmoid eye movement by simply watching the patient's eye movements often do not agree with the results of objective eye movement analysis

3. The pattern of nystagmoid eye movements cannot be used with certainty to predict the etiology of the nystagmus. Some general rules exist (e.g., early-onset nystagmus is usually horizontal), but there are exceptions

4. The same patient may exhibit different types of nystagmoid eye movements on different occasions

5. Nystagmus is often worse when the patient is under stress or tries hard to see

6. The level of visual acuity in nystagmus is only loosely correlated with the type or amplitude of nystagmoid eye movements

in Table 7.2. Early-onset nystagmus is often associated with a null zone: a direction of gaze in which the nystagmus is minimized and the vision optimized. Patients typically adopt a head position to cause them to look in this direction of gaze.

It is important to describe the characteristics of the nystagmus in clinical records, but this is difficult because it is hard to describe a form of movement in words, and the characteristics may change from one moment to another. Nonetheless, an attempt should be made and Table 7.3 describes the key features of nystagmus that can be described in clinical records.

When do I need to do something?

Most cases of nystagmus seen in primary eyecare practice are long-standing, unchanging and require no action. Any cases in which the nystagmus is of recent onset or changing require referral.

Table 7.2   Differential diagnosis of the main types of nystagmus

Early-onset nystagmus	Latent nystagmus	Acquired nystagmus
Presents in first 6 months of life	Usually presents in first 6 months of life, and almost always in first 12 months	Onset at any age and usually associated with other symptoms (e.g., nausea, vertigo, movement or balance disorders)
Family history often present	May be family history of underlying cause (e.g., infantile esotropia syndrome)	History may include head trauma or neurological disease (e.g., multiple sclerosis)
Oscillopsia absent or rare under normal viewing conditions	Oscillopsia absent or rare under normal viewing conditions	Oscillopsia common; may also have diplopia
Usually horizontal; although small vertical and torsional movements may be present. Pure vertical or torsional presentations are rare	Always horizontal; and, on monocular occlusion, saccadic, beating away from the covered eye (so direction reverses when occluder is moved from one eye to the other)	Oscillations may be horizontal, vertical, or torsional depending on the site of the lesion
The eye movements are bilateral and conjugate to the naked eye	Oscillations are always conjugate	Oscillations may be disconjugate and in different planes
May be present with other ocular conditions: albinism, achromatopsia, aniridia, optic atrophy	Usually occurs secondary to infantile esotropia syndrome; sometimes in association with DVD (p. 56)	Results from pathological lesion or trauma affecting motor areas of brain or motor pathways

(continued)

Table 7.2 **Continued**

Early-onset nystagmus	Latent nystagmus	Acquired nystagmus
A head turn may be present, usually to utilize a null zone	May be a head turn in the direction of the fixing eye	There may be a gaze direction in which nystagmus is absent, and a corresponding head turn
Intensity may lessen on convergence but it is worse when fatigued or under stress	More intense when the fixing eye abducts, less on adduction	

What do I do?

For the new or changing cases described above, the management is referral. The urgency of the referral depends on a variety of factors, most significantly the speed of onset. If a patient reports nystagmus and oscillopsia for the first time today, then very urgent referral is indicated. If their long-standing nystagmus appears to be gradually worsening over a period of several months, then non-urgent referral is indicated. It is also important to take account of the patient's general health. If this is poor, or there are other neurological signs (e.g., headache, unsteady gait), then the referral becomes more urgent.

One or two things need to be borne in mind in dealing with patients with long-standing and stable nystagmus. If they have a null position, then do not do anything to make it harder for them to use this zone. For example, if they have a null zone in upgaze and they use this when reading then bifocal or varifocal spectacles are contra-indicated. If there is a latent component (worse with monocular viewing) then monovision may be contra-indicated.

Many cases of long-standing nystagmus have quite high refractive errors and careful correction of these can help the

Table 7.3 Clinical observations of nystagmus

Characteristic	Observations
General observations	General posture, facial asymmetries, head posture
Apparent type of nystagmus	Pendular, jerk or mixed
Direction	Horizontal, vertical, torsional or combination
Amplitude	Small (<4Δ), moderate (4–20Δ), large (>20Δ)
Frequency	Slow (<0.5 cycle per second; Hz), moderate (0.5–2 Hz), fast (>2 Hz)
Constancy	Constant, intermittent, periodic
Conjugacy	Conjugate (both eyes' movements approximately parallel), disjunctive (eyes move independently) or monocular
Latent component	Does nystagmus increase or change with occlusion of one eye. If so, does it always beat away from the covered eye (pathognomonic of latent nystagmus)
Position of gaze changes	Null point: does nystagmus increase or decrease in any field of gaze or with convergence

patient to make the most of the vision that they have. If there is a latent component to the nystagmus then it is better not to occlude during the refraction. Instead, the Humphriss Immediate Contrast method can be used. There is some evidence that contact lenses, particularly gas-permeable rigid contact lenses, might help the patient to subconsciously control the nystagmus a little better.

Every now and then vision therapies or surgical treatments for nystagmus are advocated. So far, none of these has been supported by randomized controlled trials. There is a very good support group for people with nystagmus: the Nystagmus Network (www.nystagmusnet.org).

8
Accommodative anomalies

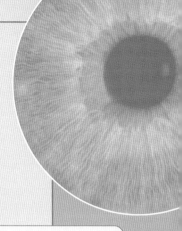

What are accommodative anomalies?

Accommodative anomalies are problems characterized by an inadequate amplitude or control of accommodation. The various types of accommodative anomaly are listed along the top row of Table 8.1 and they are fairly well defined by their clinical characteristics, also listed in Table 8.1.

How do I investigate?

The first suggestion of an accommodative problem usually comes from the patient's symptoms (Table 8.1). Careful refraction is essential, and it is usually necessary to rule out latent hypermetropia by cycloplegic refraction. Accommodative amplitude is easily measured with the push up test, typically using the RAF rule (see Table 8.2). Amplitude can also be assessed with negative lenses, although this method gives different results to the push up test.

Accommodative facility (the rate at which the accommodation can be changed) is usually measured with flippers (Figure 8.1). The procedure for this test is described in Table 8.3. The range of responses at this test in a typical population is very wide (Table 8.3) and this makes results difficult to interpret. Undoubtedly, one reason for this is that the test is very subjective. In view of the variability of the test, it is unwise to base a treatment on this test result alone, unless the symptoms are strongly suggestive of accommodative infacility.

It is usual for accommodation to lag a little behind the target, but only by 0.50–0.75D so that the target does not appear significantly blurred. Accommodative lag can be assessed by dynamic retinoscopy and this is the only routine clinical test that can be used to assess accommodative function objectively. It is an extremely useful test, especially with children where a visual conversion (hysterical) reaction is suspected. There are two main approaches to measuring the accommodative lag by retinoscopy. One of these, MEM retinoscopy, is described in Table 8.4. The idea

Table 8.1 The four main types of accommodative anomaly and their symptoms and clinical signs

	Accommodative insufficiency	Accommodative infacility	Accommodative fatigue	Accommodative spasm (excess)
Symptoms	Near blur	Difficulty changing focus (e.g., copying from board)	Near blur towards end of day	Transient blur of distance or near vision
Accommodative amplitude (Table 8.2)	Low	Normal	Declines with repeat testing	Normal
Accommodative facility (Table 8.3)	May be slow with minus lenses	Poor	Declines with repeat testing	May be slow with plus lenses
Accommodative lag (Table 8.4)	Need high plus (>+0.75)	Normal	Initially OK, increasing plus after much near vision	Need negative lenses

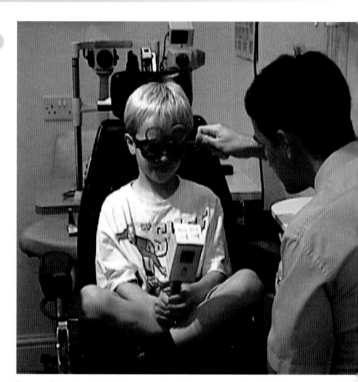

Figure 8.1 A child being tested with accommodative flippers

behind the test is that it simulates the normal situation when reading and, because the lens is only present briefly and in front of one eye, the accommodation does not relax by the power of the lens. So, the lens power that is required to neutralize the reflex is a true reflection of the accommodative lag.

Accommodative anomalies quite commonly occur in conjunction with other binocular vision anomalies, so a full eye examination is essential to fully understand the problem. In particular, combined convergence and accommodative insufficiency is quite a common condition and can be treated with eye exercises or, in intractable cases, with spectacles.

Another condition which sometimes occurs is **spasm of the near reflex**. This is characterized by an intermittent spasm of

Table 8.2 Norms for the amplitude of accommodation as measured by the push up test. Minimum normal values are given in diopters (D) and centimeters (cm)

Age (yrs)	Minimum (D)	Minimum (cm)
4	14.00	7.00
6	13.50	7.50
8	13.00	7.75
10	12.50	8.00
12	12.00	8.25
14	11.50	8.75
20	10.00	10.00
30	7.50	13.25
40	5.00	20.00
50	2.50	40.00

convergence, accommodation and pupillary miosis. Parents might report an intermittent esotropia in conjunction with a small pupil and the child may report blurred vision together with diplopia. This can be linked to a variety of neurogenic and psychogenic conditions, so referral to exclude these conditions is advisable. If these are excluded, then treatment with exercises or glasses can be helpful.

When do I need to do something?

Patients who have the symptoms and signs of an accommodative anomaly (Table 8.1) require treatment, once other causes have been excluded. Other causes of their symptoms and signs will generally be excluded by a routine eye examination. Particular care should be taken to look for signs of nervous system pathology (for example, see Table 3.3).

Table 8.3 Procedure for testing accommodative facility with flippers

1. Usually, ±2.00D lenses are used, although ±1.50 or ±1.00 can be used if the ±2.00 cannot be cleared

2. Start with the plus lenses, explaining to the patient that they have to report when the target becomes clear and single

3. The best target is one that can be used to control for suppression, such as the OXO target that is designed to test for vertical fixation disparity
   - In facility testing, this target is used simply for the child to report if they experience suppression, when one of the green strips will disappear
   - The child will need to wear polarized filters
   - The use of this target means that the patient has to report not just when the OXO becomes clear and single, but also when both green strips are present
   - For some children, this makes the test too complicated, in which case the test might have to be carried out without checking for suppression

4. As soon as the target is described as clear and single with no suppression, flip the lenses to the pair of minus lenses. Ask the child to again report when the target is clear, single and both strips are present

5. Repeat 4, flipping to the plus lenses

6. Continue, measuring how many cycles can be completed in 1 minute (cycles per minute; cpm). Note that one cycle is two flips

7. The binocular list norms are that about 90% of the population perform better than 2 cpm and about 50% of the population perform better than 7 cpm. If there is an abnormal test result binocularly, the test can be repeated monocularly

If the visual acuity is normal at distance but abnormal at near then this supports the diagnosis of an accommodative anomaly. As mentioned above, latent hypermetropia needs to be excluded and the usual way of doing this is to carry out a cycloplegic refraction.

Table 8.4 **Procedure for measuring accommodative lag with MEM retinoscopy**

1.	The retinoscopy is carried out at the patient's usual reading distance
2.	The patient wears any refractive correction that they usually use for reading
3.	The patient fixates a target on the retinoscope. Because the target is in the plane of the retinoscope, no correction needs to be made for working distance
4.	The target is viewed binocularly, although the retinoscopy is of course only carried out on one eye at a time
5.	Retinoscopy is usually only carried out in the horizontal meridian
6.	Typically a "with" movement is seen indicating that the accommodation is lagging behind the target (plus lenses need to be added). An "against" movement suggests accommodative spasm (see Table 8.1)
7.	Spherical lenses are introduced of a power that it is thought will neutralize the reflex. For a typical "with" movement, the first lens might be +0.50
8.	The lens is introduced monocularly and is rapidly interposed: it should be present for no more than $^1/_2$ second. This should be just long enough for a "sweep" of the retinoscope to see if the reflex is now neutralized
9.	If the reflex is not neutralized, then steps 7–8 are repeated until the reflex is neutralized
10.	Steps 4–9 are then repeated for the other eye
11.	The normal range of response (mean $\pm$ 1SD) is plano to +0.75D

What do I do?

A sudden-onset marked decrease in the amplitude of accommodation can be a sign of accommodative paralysis, which can result from neurological pathology. Such cases should be

Table 8.5 Treatments for accommodative anomalies

	Accommodative insufficiency	Accommodative infacility	Accommodative fatigue	Accommodative spasm (excess)
Eye exercises	Push up exercises	Facility exercises	Push up or flippers	Distance to near or flipper or push up
Refractive	Plus lenses or multifocals	If severe, multifocals	Plus lenses or multifocals	Rarely multifocals

referred. In other less acute and milder cases of accommodative anomalies, where there are no suspicious signs (for example, exclude the signs in Table 3.3), the patient can be treated but should be carefully monitored to make sure that the condition does not deteriorate. Treatments are outlined in Table 8.5. A letter of information to the general practitioner is advisable in case the patient presents to them with any other symptoms which, together with the accommodative anomaly, might raise the index of suspicion of pathology.

Index

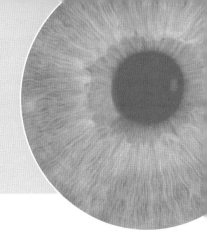